FOGSI Focus
Genetics for the Generalist

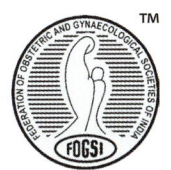 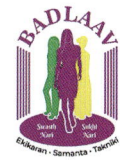

FOGSI Focus
Genetics for the Generalist

Series Editor
Hrishikesh D Pai
MD FRCOG (UK-HON) FCPS FICOG MSc (USA)
President, FOGSI (Federation of Obstetric and Gynaecological Societies of India)
Professor
Department of Reproductive Medicine
DY Patil University, Navi Mumbai
Founder and Medical Director
Bloom IVF Group, Mumbai
Consultant Gynecologist
Lilavati Hospital IVF Centre, Mumbai
Fortis, New Delhi and Chandigarh
Hospital Bloom IVF Centre
Mumbai, Maharashtra, India

Editors
Seetha Ramamurthy Pal
MBBS DGO MD MRCOG FICOG RCOG/RCR Diploma in Obst USG
Consultant
Department of Obstetrics and Fetal Medicine
Apollo Multispecialty Hospitals
Kolkata, West Bengal, India
Chair, Genetics and Fetal Medicine Committee, FOGSI

Vandana Bansal
MD DGO DNB MNAMS FICOG FRCOG (UK) FNB (High Risk Pregnancy and Perinatology)
Additional Professor
Nowrosjee Wadia Maternity Hospital and GS Medical College, Mumbai
Director, Fetal Medicine Centre
Surya Mother and Child Hospital
Mumbai, Maharashtra, India

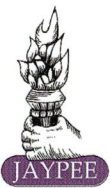

JAYPEE BROTHERS MEDICAL PUBLISHERS
The Health Sciences Publisher
New Delhi | London

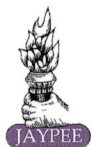
Jaypee Brothers Medical Publishers (P) Ltd.

Headquarters
Jaypee Brothers Medical Publishers (P) Ltd
EMCA House, 23/23-B
Ansari Road, Daryaganj
New Delhi 110 002, India
Landline: +91-11-23272143, +91-11-23272703
+91-11-23282021, +91-11-23245672
Email: jaypee@jaypeebrothers.com

Corporate Office
Jaypee Brothers Medical Publishers (P) Ltd
4838/24, Ansari Road, Daryaganj
New Delhi 110 002, India
Phone: +91-11-43574357
Fax: +91-11-43574314
Email: jaypee@jaypeebrothers.com

Overseas Office
JP Medical Ltd.
83, Victoria Street, London
SW1H 0HW (UK)
Phone: +44 20 3170 8910
Fax: +44 (0)20 3008 6180
Email: info@jpmedpub.com

Website: www.jaypeebrothers.com
Website: www.jaypeedigital.com

© 2024, Jaypee Brothers Medical Publishers

The views and opinions expressed in this book are solely those of the original contributor(s)/author(s) and do not necessarily represent those of editor(s) or publisher of the book.

All rights reserved. No part of this publication may be reproduced, stored or transmitted in any form or by any means, electronic, mechanical, photocopying, recording or otherwise, without the prior permission in writing of the publishers.

All brand names and product names used in this book are trade names, service marks, trademarks or registered trademarks of their respective owners. The publisher is not associated with any product or vendor mentioned in this book.

Medical knowledge and practice change constantly. This book is designed to provide accurate, authoritative information about the subject matter in question. However, readers are advised to check the most current information available on procedures included and check information from the manufacturer of each product to be administered, to verify the recommended dose, formula, method and duration of administration, adverse effects and contraindications. It is the responsibility of the practitioner to take all appropriate safety precautions. Neither the publisher nor the author(s)/editor(s) assume any liability for any injury and/or damage to persons or property arising from or related to use of material in this book.

This book is sold on the understanding that the publisher is not engaged in providing professional medical services. If such advice or services are required, the services of a competent medical professional should be sought.

Every effort has been made where necessary to contact holders of copyright to obtain permission to reproduce copyright material. If any have been inadvertently overlooked, the publisher will be pleased to make the necessary arrangements at the first opportunity.

Inquiries for bulk sales may be solicited at: jaypee@jaypeebrothers.com

FOGSI Focus: Genetics for the Generalist

First Edition: **2024**

ISBN: 978-93-5696-987-2

Printed at: Samrat Offset Pvt. Ltd.

Dedicated to

The women of India

CONTRIBUTORS

Debasmita Mandal
MBBS MD (Obs & Gyne) FICOG FIAOG
Director
Krishnaya Institute of Cardiac and Fetal Sciences
Kolkata, West Bengal, India

Deepti Gupta MBBS MS DNB FICOG
Associate Professor
Department of Obstetrics and Gynecology
NSCB Medical College, Jabalpur
Consultant and Unit Head
Ankur Fertility Clinic and IVF Centre
Jabalpur, Madhya Pradesh, India

Dipanjana Datta PhD PDF (USA)
Consultant Genetic Counselor
Renew Healthcare
Apollo Multispecialty Hospitals
Institute of Fetal Medicine
Bhagirathi Neotia Woman and Child Care Centre
Kolkata, West Bengal, India

Dpankar Banerji MBBS MS
Consultant and Unit Head
Ideal Fertility Center
Jabalpur, Madhya Pradesh, India

Jyotshna Rani Panigrahi
MBBS MD (Obs & Gyne) Fellow in Fetal Medicine (Hons & Gold Medalist)
Director
Mom and Childcare Fetal Medicine Centre
Cuttack, Odisha, India

Malathi G Prasad
MD FRCOG (UK) Diploma in Fetal Medicine (FMF Barcelona)
Lead Fetal Medicine Consultant
Trichy Fetal Medicine Centre
Tiruchirappalli, Tamil Nadu, India

Meenakshi Lallar
MBBS MS DM (Medical Genetics)
Consultant Clinical Geneticist
Prime Diagnostics, Chandigarh
Consultant Clinical Geneticist
MedGenome Labs
Bengaluru, Karnataka, India

Meera Jayaprakash
MS (Obs & Gyne) FCPS Fellowship in Fetal Medicine (MUHS)
Consultant
Siddhivinayak Hospital
Bhandara, Maharashtra, India

Megha Kamalapurkar MD
Consultant, Obstetrician and Gynecologist
Devata Hospital
Kalaburagi, Karnataka, India

Megha Sharma
MBBS MS DNB PDCC (High Risk Pregnancy & Fetal Medicine)
Consultant
Nidaan Heart and Fetal Medicine Clinic
Kota, Rajasthan, India

Rekha Gupta
MBBS MS DM (Medical Genetics)
Assistant Professor
Department of Medical Genetics
Mahatma Gandhi Medical College
Jaipur, Rajasthan, India

Safa Abdul Syed Basheerudeen
BSc (Microbiology) MSc (Molecular Biology) PhD (Radiation Genetics)
Senior Scientist
Microbiological Laboratory,
Molecular and Genomic Centre
Tiruchirappalli, Tamil Nadu, India

Saswati Mukhopadhyay
DNB (Obs & Gyne) DrNB (Medical Genetics)
Consultant Clinical Geneticist
Apollo Multispecialty Hospital
Kolkata, West Bengal, India

Seetha Ramamurthy Pal
MBBS DGO MD MRCOG FICOG RCOG/RCR Diploma in Obst USG
Consultant
Department of Obstetrics and Fetal Medicine
Apollo Multispecialty Hospitals
Kolkata, West Bengal, India
Chair, Genetics and Fetal Medicine Committee, FOGSI

Shovandeb Kalapahar MS DNB FNB
Consultant
Department of Reproductive Medicine
Institute of Reproductive Medicine
Kolkata, West Bengal, India

Shruti Jain
MBBS MS DNB PDCC (Maternal and Fetal Medicine)
Consultant Fetal Medicine
Kailash Hospital
Noida, Uttar Pradesh, India

Shyama Devadasan
MS (Obs & Gyne) Fellowship in Feto–Maternal Medicine
Chief Consultant in Fetal Medicine
Ambady Scan Centre, Thrissur
Visiting Consultant
Apollo Adlux Hospital, Angamaly
Pran Fertility and Well Woman Centre
Thiruvananthapuram, Kerala, India

Sujoy Dasgupta MS DNB MRCOG MSc
Consultant
Department of Reproductive Medicine
Genome Fertility Centre
Kolkata, West Bengal, India

Suma Vishnu
MBBS MS DNB (OBG) Fellowship in
Advanced Obstetric Ultrasound
Consultant
Department of Obstetrics and
Gynecology
Vinayaka Hospital
Wayanad, Kerala, India

Vaishnavi PK
MBBS MS (OBG) Fellowship in Feto-Maternal
Medicine (RGUHS)
Consultant in Obstetrics and
Gynecology
Clinic for Women
Bengaluru, Karnataka, India

Vandana Bansal
MD DGO DNB MNAMS FICOG FRCOG (UK)
FNB (High Risk Pregnancy and Perinatology)
Additional Professor
Nowrosjee Wadia Maternity Hospital
and GS Medical College, Mumbai
Director, Fetal Medicine Centre
Surya Mother and Child Hospital
Mumbai, Maharashtra, India

OFFICE BEARERS OF TEAM FOGSI 2023

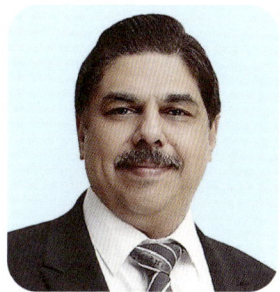
Dr Hrishikesh D Pai
President

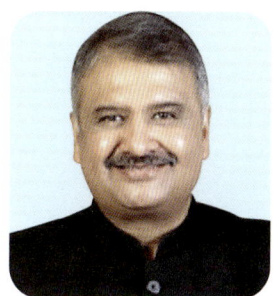
Dr Jaydeep Tank
President Elect

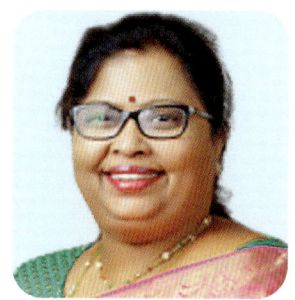
Dr S Shantha Kumari
Immediate Past President

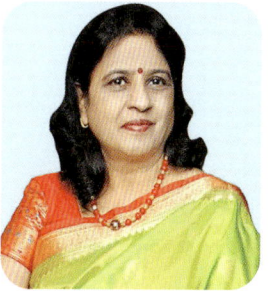
Dr Madhuri Patel
Secretary General

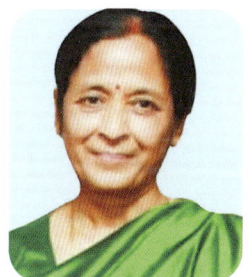
Dr Alka Pandey
Vice President

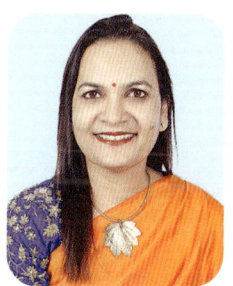
Dr Asha Baxi
Vice President

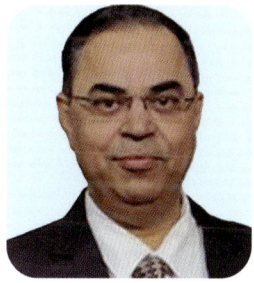
Dr Geetendra Sharma
Vice President

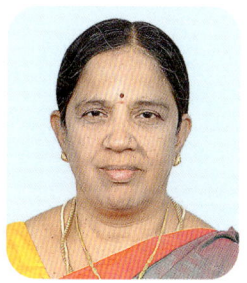
Dr S Sampathkumari
Vice President

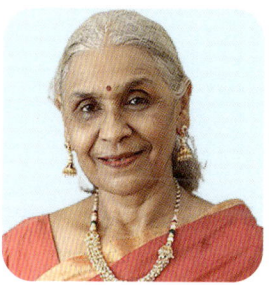
Dr Yashodhara Pradeep
Vice President

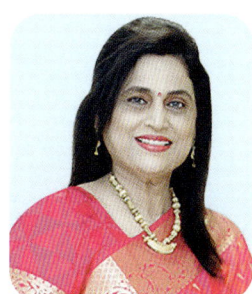
Dr Suvarna Khadilkar
Dp Secretary General

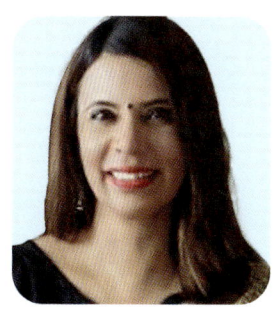
Dr Manisha Takhtani
Joint Secretary

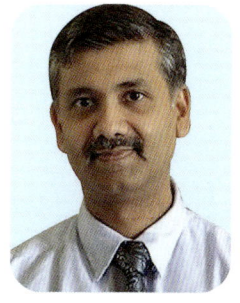
Dr Parikshit Tank
Treasurer

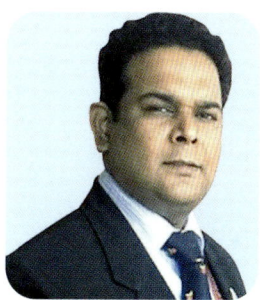
Dr Niranjan Chavan
Joint Treasurer

FROM THE PRESIDENT'S DESK

Dear Fogsians,
Greetings!!

It gives me immense pleasure to bring to you this FOGSI Focus on "Genetics for the Generalists".

The field of genetics has increased dramatically in last few decades, and we as obstetrician and gynecologists are increasingly called on to incorporate genetics and genetic testing in our day-to-day practice. This focus is a crisp compilation of chapters focusing on the role of genetics in pregnancy and different gynecological problems and infertility. The chapters are in the form of simple algorithms with stress on main key points thereby making it easier for readers to understand and apply the same in routine practice.

FOGSI has always played a vital role in spreading the knowledge both among doctors and patients. This year my FOGSI slogan is *Swasthya Nari, Sukhi Nari*. My CSR activity is defined as *Badlaav* (Change) including three arms- *Ekikaran* (integration of thought and action), *Samanta* (equality of treatment irrespective of economic status) and *Takniki* (technology to achieve these objectives). These academic publications are a step towards my goal of improving women's health in our country, by providing updated information about the relevant topics in women care.

It will be a ready reckoner for both the students and clinicians to update their knowledge on evidence-based management. I congratulate Dr Seetha Ramamurthy Pal and all the editors and co-editors for their sincere efforts to write, collate, edit and publish this Focus.

I sincerely hope that this focus will benefit and empower all the FOGSIANS.

Wish you all a happy reading!!

Hrishikesh D Pai
President, FOGSI (2022–2023)

PREFACE

We are currently living in the era of genomic revolution and clinical genetics is one of the most rapidly advancing fields in medicine. A lot of progress and advances have been achieved in the field of genetics, especially in screening, prenatal diagnosis of genetic disorders and genetic evaluations in gynecology. Diagnosing a genetic disorder not only allows for disease specific management options but also has implications for the affected individual's entire family. Medicine is undergoing a paradigm shift with genetics being incorporated in every aspect of patient management. Hence a working understanding of the underlying concepts of genetic diseases, tests used, and their significance is important for all practicing clinicians.

Through this FOGSI Focus, my Co-editor and I have tried to bring an updated ready-reckoner of essentials in genetics which is basically Genetics for the Generalist. We sincerely hope that this focus will be useful and simple and help our FOGSIans to incorporate genetics in their daily practice.

Seetha Ramamurthy Pal
Vandana Bansal

ACKNOWLEDGMENTS

As the Chairperson of the Genetics and Fetal Medicine Committee, FOGSI, I would like to thank our visionary and dynamic President, FOGSI, Dr Hrishikesh D Pai, for giving me the opportunity to come out with the FOGSI Focus on Genetics for the Generalist. I would also like to express my gratitude to our Secretary General, Dr Madhuri Patel, for her guidance always.

It is my proud privilege to thank my Co-editor, Dr Vandana Bansal, who has assisted me in reviewing the chapters and for her expert inputs in compiling it. I also sincerely thank all the contributors who despite their busy schedule have given their valuable time and input in making this Focus so simple and lucid. Last but not least, I am thankful to M/s Jaypee Brothers Medical Publishers (P) Ltd, New Delhi, India, for their efforts in bringing out this book.

Seetha Ramamurthy Pal

CONTENTS

1. Basics of Genetics 1
Seetha Ramamurthy Pal
- Genome *1*; • Chromosome *1*; • Deoxyribonucleic Acid *2*; • Genes *2*

2. Pedigree Charting 5
Megha Sharma, Rekha Gupta
- Autosomal Dominant *5*; • Autosomal Recessive *7*; • X-linked Dominant *7*; • X-linked Recessive *7*
- Y-linked Disorders *9*; • Mitochondrial Inheritance *9*

3. Carrier Screening and Genetic Inheritance 10
Malathi G Prasad, Safa Abdul Syed Basheerudeen
- Genetic Carrier Testing/Screening *10*; • Genetic Inheritance Pattern *10*; • Types of Genetic Tests *11*
- The American College of Obstetricians and Gynecologists Recommendations *12*

4. Preconception Genetic Counseling 14
Deepti Gupta, Dpankar Banerji
- Definition *14*; • Risk Assessment *14*; • Genetic Testing *15*; • Pretest Counseling *15*
- Post-test Counseling *16*

5. Genetic Tests and their Significance in Prenatal Evaluation 17
Shyama Devadasan
- Noninvasive Prenatal Screening *17*; • Diagnostic Procedures *17*
- Indications of Prenatal Genetic Testing *19*; • Types of Genetic Tests *19*

6. Genetic Counseling in Cases of Abnormal Serum Screening 22
Suma Vishnu
- Serum Screening *22*; • Types of Screening Tests *23*; • Second Trimester *23*; • Counseling *23*
- Interpretation of Results *23*; • Diagnostic Testing *24*

7. Genetics and Counseling in Hemoglobinopathies 27
Megha Kamalapurkar, Vaishnavi PK
- Incidence *27*; • Normal Hemoglobin *27*; • Classification *27*
- Screening of Hemoglobinopathies *29*; • How to do Screening? *29*

8. Common Congenital Fetal Anomalies and Genetic Associations 32
Vandana Bansal, Meera Jayaprakash
- First Trimester Nuchal Translucency and Anomaly Scan *32*; • Second Trimester Genetic Sonogram *33*
- Second Trimester Structural Anomalies and Association with Genetic Abnormalities *34*
- Central Nervous System *36*; • Fetal Face *38*; • Fetal Abdomen *38*
- Congenital Lung Malformations *39*; • Fetal Gastrointestinal Anomalies *40*
- Skeletal System *40*; • Fetal Genitourinary Anomalies *40*; • Fetal Heart *41*

9. Genetics and Infertility 46
Shovandeb Kalapahar, Sujoy Dasgupta
- Genetics in Female Infertility *46*; • Genetics of Male Infertility *48*
- Genetics for Preimplantation Genetic Testing *50*

10. Genetics and Recurrent Pregnancy Loss 53
Debasmita Mandal, Jyotshna Rani Panigrahi
- Aneuploidy *53*; • Translocation *54*; • Copy Number Variations *54*
- Mosaicism *54*; • Mutations and Single Nucleic Variations *54*
- Epigenetic Studies *55*; • Evaluation of Products of Conception *56*
- Management Options for Genetic Issues of Recurrent Pregnancy Loss *56*

11. Preimplantation Genetic Diagnosis 58
Dipanjana Datta
- Process Development and Testing Platforms for Preimplantation Genetic Testing *58*
- Indications for Preimplantation Genetic Testing *59*; • Why is it A Screening Test? *60*

12. Genetics and Inherited Cancers 62
Saswati Mukhopadhyay
- Mechanisms of Hereditary Cancer Predisposition *62*
- Major Types of Hereditary Cancer Syndromes *63*; • Management of Hereditary Tumors *64*

13. Gene Therapy 66
Shruti Jain, Meenakshi Lallar
- Types of Gene Therapy *66*; • In Utero Gene Therapy *66*; • Strategies of Gene Therapy *67*
- Approach to Gene Therapy *67*; • Methods of Gene Delivery *67*; • History of Gene Therapy *67*
- Challenges with Gene Therapy *68*

Index *71*

Chapter 1

Basics of Genetics

Seetha Ramamurthy Pal

■ INTRODUCTION

Genetics is the study of genetic traits that an individual possesses and how these traits are passed from one generation to another. With increasing knowledge of the molecular basis of inherited disorders and the advances in the development of various deoxyribonucleic acid (DNA) based tests, it has now become possible to diagnose many of these conditions prenatally and postnatally, do carrier testing in affected families and screen for aneuploidy effectively. As a result, it has become necessary for every healthcare provider to incorporate genetics and genetic testing in their day-to-day practice.

■ GENOME

The entire genetic material in a chromosome set is called the genome **(Fig. 1)**. The identification and mapping of the full human DNA sequence was completed in 2003 as part of the Human Genome Project.[1] This project produced a detailed map of the genes and other important areas along each chromosome.

Every human cell has a nucleus and each nucleus contains 23 pairs of chromosomes inherited from each parent, in which 22 pairs are numbered chromosomes called autosomes and one pair called sex chromosomes, designated as X and Y chromosomes.

■ CHROMOSOME

Each chromosome is composed of multiple long linear DNA molecules in a complex with large variety of proteins called histone in a double helix shape. Histones are the packaging proteins which bind the DNA molecules and condense it to maintain its integrity. It provides

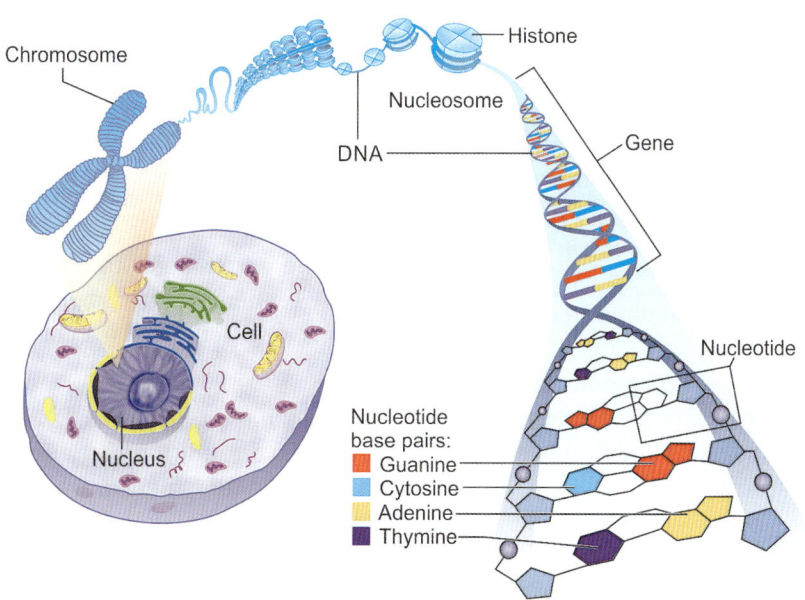

Fig. 1: Deoxyribonucleic acid (DNA) structure.

structural support to the chromosome and gives a more compact three-dimensional structure. During metaphase of mitosis, the duplicated chromosomes are joined by a central strand is composed mere, resulting in an X-shaped structure. This is highly condensed and normally visible under a light microscope which can be counted and thus easiest to distinguish for chromosome analysis. The chromosome constitution of an individual is known as the karyotype.

■ DEOXYRIBONUCLEIC ACID

Deoxyribonucleic acid is a molecule that carries genetic information of all living cells. It consists of two strands wind around one another to form a double helix. Each strand is made of alternating sugars (deoxyribose) and phosphate groups and one of the four bases—adenine, cytosine, guanine and thymine attached to each sugar molecule in various combinations. The most common methods of DNA extraction are phenol/chloroform extraction methods which isolate DNAs from proteins. After the DNA is extracted, it can be analyzed by restriction fragment length polymorphism or qualitative analysis by polymerase chain reaction to diagnose any disease.

■ GENES

The DNA includes approximately 25,000–30,000 genes. A gene is a segment of DNA that directs synthesis of one or more molecules of proteins that help the body carry out various functions. Each gene is a unique series of four nucleotides that ultimately codes for an amino acid sequence that is needed to form a protein. The coding regions in the genes are called *exons* which are DNA sequences that will be transcribed into messenger RNA (mRNA—messenger ribonucleic acid) and the noncoding areas are the *introns*. Each pair of chromosomes contains the same genes, but they may have different versions of those genes as we inherit one chromosome in each pair from our mother and father.

Approximately, 1.5% of the genome is composed of exons which are collectively called the exome.

The whole structure can be compared to a book where the genome is the book, the chromosomes are the chapters, the genes are the sentences, and the nucleotides are the letters.

Terminologies

Genotype: This refers to the genetic material passed between generations.

Phenotype: This is the physical appearance or traits seen in an individual that results from the expression of the genotype and its interaction with the environment. Each autosomal gene has an influence in determining the phenotype and this is described as dominant or recessive.

Alleles: These are normal variants within the population. The genes that determine blood group and Rhesus factor have several normal alleles. The exact position on the chromosome that contains a particular gene is called the locus. Humans inherit two copies of the same allele, which is said to be homozygous or two different alleles when it is called heterozygous for that locus.

Polymorphisms: Most DNA is identical among all humans. Polymorphisms are small differences in the DNA and they usually consist of single nucleotide polymorphisms, deletions, or duplications that occur every 200–500 base pairs. In most cases, these polymorphisms are benign variants and do not cause disease but sometimes they may modify the gene function and cause disease.

Pathogenic variant: Also known as mutation, this is an alteration in the DNA sequence which causes change in the protein structure or function resulting in adverse effects.

The American College of Medical Genetics has defined a classification system for variants—pathogenic, likely pathogenic, benign, likely benign, and uncertain significance.[2] When these variants occur in the germline (gametes), they are likely to be transmitted from one generation to the next but when they occur in the somatic cells, they are more likely to be associated with cancer.

When an identified DNA change cannot be reliably characterized as benign or pathogenic, it is referred to as variant of uncertain significance.

The types of variants are as follows:[3]

Single nucleotide variant (SNV): As the name suggests, when there are changes to a single nucleotide within the DNA sequence, such as single base substitutions, insertions, or deletions, it is known as single nucleotide variant.

Deletions and duplications: Deletion of a genomic information or addition can affect the gene function. Both very small (single nucleotide) and very large (entire chromosome) deletions and insertions of genetic information can impact the gene function.

Indel (insertion/deletion) is the term currently used for deletions and duplications of <1 kb.

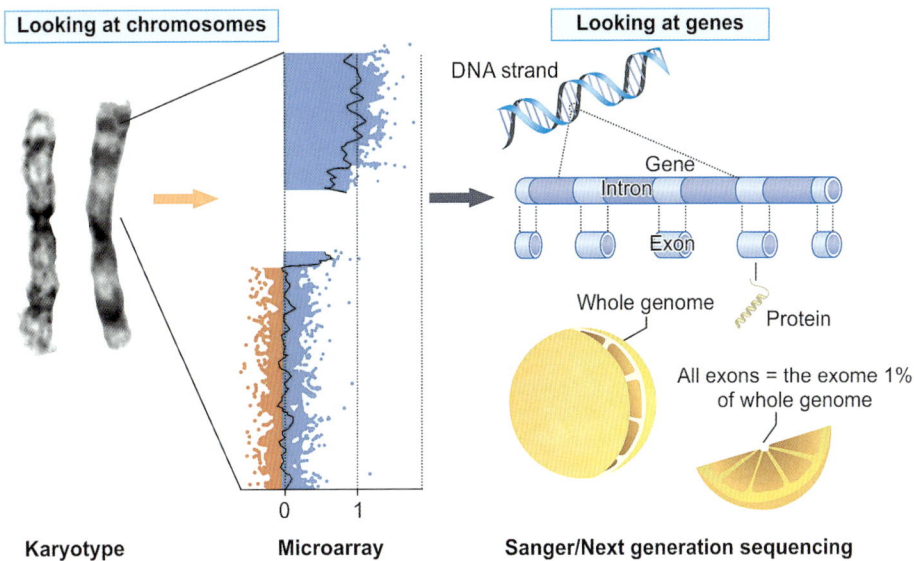

Fig. 2: Diagnostic capability of genetic tests.

Copy number variation (CNV) is typically used for deletions and duplications of >1 kb. This can involve an entire chromosome like in trisomy 21.

Trinucleotide repeat expansion: This is a type of duplication where three specific nucleotides recur multiple times in a row and cause a change in the function of the protein, for example, Friedreich's ataxia.

Methylation: The addition of methyl groups to DNA can make the gene inactive and the changes that occur in the methylation pattern can cause disease. It is important to note that these changes do not affect the DNA sequence.

Mitochondrial variants: Mitochondrial DNA is a special type of DNA present in the mitochondria and its main characteristic is that this DNA is always maternally inherited. This is passed entirely unchanged through the maternal line and cannot pass through males. Changes in the mitochondrial DNA can lead to cell malfunctioning or cellular death altogether resulting in severe organ dysfunction.

Penetrance: It is the proportion of individuals carrying a particular variant of a gene that also expresses an associated trait. This can be either complete penetrance when there is phenotypic expression in all individuals or incomplete penetrance where the gene is not fully expressed in all individuals.

Expressivity: It is the extent to which a phenotype is expressed by individuals having a particular genotype. This can be full, moderate, mild, or variable.

Pleiotropy: When a single gene mutation causes multiple traits in an individual, it is known as pleiotropy such as the β-globin gene mutation affecting various organ functions.

Mosaicism: The presence of two or more cell lines with different characteristics within one organ or tissue. This can be either germline mosaicism, which is the result of sporadic mutation in a cell that will give rise to a gamete cell or somatic mosaicism is the accumulation of mutations in DNA sequence in cellular genomes after fertilization.

Epigenetics: Epigenetics describes a process by which genes can be modified biochemically and this can affect the gene expression without actually changing the DNA sequence. They can be affected by developmental factors, environmental chemicals, drugs, aging, and diet.

Imprinting: This is a mechanism where epigenetic control of genetic expression occurs and the extent of imprinting is determined by the sex of the transmitting parent.

Depending on the pathology, various tests can be used. The tests can be broadly divided into two types of tests that firstly assess chromosomal variants such as karyotype analysis and chromosomal microarray and secondly detect sequence variants such as condition-specific tests, targeted mutation analysis, broad multigene testing, whole exome, or whole genome analysis **(Fig. 2)**.[4]

■ CONCLUSION

As human genetics becomes an integral part of our daily practice, it is important for all healthcare providers to be aware of the basics and advancements in the understanding of genetics and genetic diseases. This will help in counseling patients about genetic conditions, their significance and the appropriate test that needs to be done in detecting these conditions and also to refer to genetic professionals when necessary.

REFERENCES

1. National Human Genome Research Institute. The Human Genome Project. [online] Available from: https://www.genome.gov/human-genome-project [Last accessed September, 2023].
2. Richards S, Aziz N, Bale S, Bick D, Das S, Gastier-Foster J, et al. Standards and guidelines for the interpretation of sequence variants: a joint consensus recommendation of the American College of Medical Genetics and Genomics and the Association for Molecular Pathology. Genet Med. 2015;17:405-24.
3. ACOG Technology Assessment in Obstetrics and Gynecology No. 14 Summary: Modern Genetics in Obstetrics and Gynecology. Obstet Gynecol. 2018;132(3):807-8.
4. Malhotra N, Arora V, Malhotra N, Malhotra J, Malhotra K. Genetics for the obstetrician and gynaecologists. J South Asian Feder Obst Gynae. 2023;15(2):217-25.

Chapter 2

Pedigree Charting

Megha Sharma, Rekha Gupta

◼ INTRODUCTION

A pedigree is a pictorial representation of a family tree using standard symbols. It is a chart that depicts graphically the inheritance of a trait or health condition through generations of a family, which makes it easy to understand and interpret. Thus, it can prove as an easy tool for understanding the pattern of inheritance of a particular disorder/trait and thereby helps in counseling and planning of future conceptions.

The pedigree of at least three generations is essential to arrive at any fruitful conclusion.

Analysis of the pedigree is done using the principles of Mendelian inheritance.

A standard set of symbols is used globally for pedigree charting, with minor differences amongst various genetic counseling centers and practitioners, thus standardizing the method **(Figs. 1A and B)**.

- Males are represented as squares, while females are represented as circles.
- The female is shown on the right of the male in mating pairs.
- A horizontal line between man and woman represents mating and resulting children are shown as offshoots to this line.
- Offspring are depicted from left to right in descending order of age and denoted by Arabic numerals.
- The affected member, through whom a family with a genetic disorder is brought to attention, is the *proband*.[1] The person (family member) who seeks genetic counseling is referred to as *consultand*.[2]
- Shaded symbols mean an individual is affected by a condition, while an unshaded symbol means they are unaffected.
- Generations are labelled with roman numerals.
- Members of the same generation are placed at the same horizontal level.
- If the sex of the person is unknown a diamond symbol is used.
- Heterozygotes, or carriers, when identifiable, are indicated by a shade dot inside a symbol or a half-filled symbol.
- For pregnancies not carried till term, the symbols are smaller and the line is shorter. The gestational age and gender are written below if known **(Fig. 2)**.
- *Obligate heterozygote:* An individual who must be heterozygous for a variant based on analysis of the family history; applies to disorders inherited in an autosomal recessive or X-linked manner. The term "obligate heterozygote" can also refer to individuals with an autosomal dominant disorder whose position in a pedigree indicates that they must be heterozygous even though they do not manifest the phenotype.

Once a pedigree is charted using standard symbols and using accurate information, the patterns of inheritance can be determined. There are six possible patterns of inheritance

1. Autosomal dominant
2. Autosomal recessive
3. X-linked dominant
4. X-linked recessive
5. Y-linked disorders
6. Mitochondrial inheritance.

◼ AUTOSOMAL DOMINANT

Autosomal dominant disorders manifest when only one of the two parental genes is mutated. That parent may or may not express the disorder based on variable expressivity and penetrance.

The same genetic variant found in different individuals can cause a range of diverse phenotypes, from no discernible clinical phenotype to severe disease, even among related individuals. Such variants can be said to

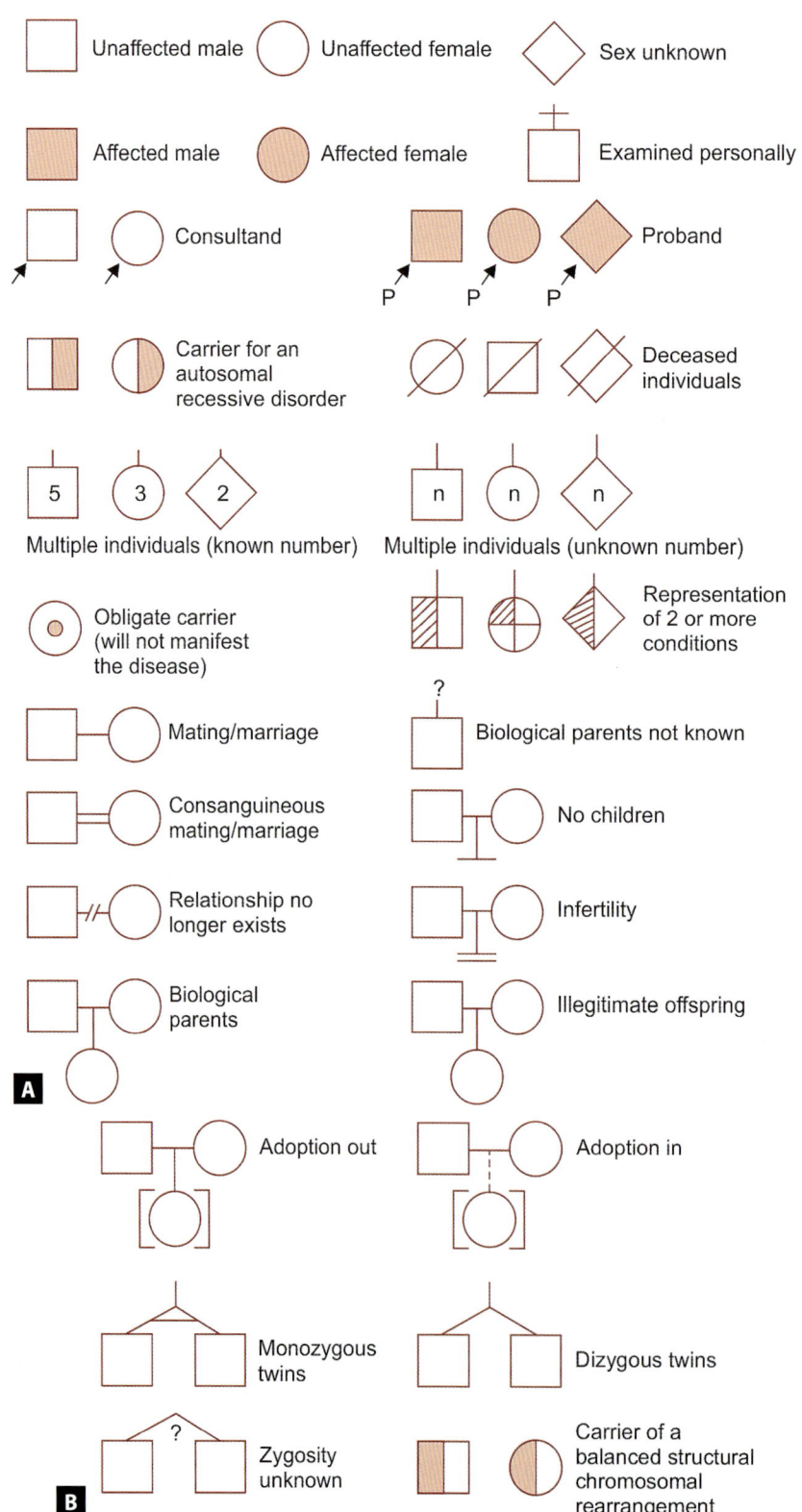

Figs. 1A and B: Standard pedigree symbols.
Source: Adapted from "Phadke SR. Genetics for Clinicians. Prism Publications; 2006."[1]

display incomplete penetrance, a binary phenomenon where the genotype either causes the expected clinical phenotype or it does not, or they can be said to display variable expressivity, in which the same genotype can cause a wide range of clinical symptoms across a spectrum. Both incomplete penetrance and variable expressivity are thought to be caused by a range of factors, including common variants, variants in regulatory regions, epigenetics, environmental factors, and lifestyle.[3]

Both males and females are equally affected.

Both males and females can transmit the disease to their offspring of either sex.

The risk of transmission of the disease from an affected parent to his or her children is 50% **(Fig. 3)**.

They may also occur as a de novo mutation in a single generation, with nonaffected parents.

Examples: Huntington's disease, Marfan syndrome, and achondroplasia.

■ AUTOSOMAL RECESSIVE

Autosomal recessive disorders manifest when both parents' genes are mutated for the particular disease. Both parents are carriers for the disorder. The parents can be consanguineous, especially if the disorder is rare. However, consanguinity is not essential.

Both males and females are affected.

The disorder normally occurs in only one generation.

The risk of transmission or having an affected child is 25% **(Fig. 4)**.

If a carrier of an autosomal recessive disorder marries an affected person, 50% of the children will be affected and the pedigree will resemble that of an autosomal dominant disorder. This is known as *pseudodominance*.

Examples: Cystic fibrosis, beta thalassemia major, sickle cell anemias, and Tay–Sachs disease.

■ X-LINKED DOMINANT

Both males and females can be affected; females are less severely affected than males.

Affected males pass on the disease to all the daughters, but none to the sons.

Affected females can pass on the disease to both daughters and sons.

There is no male-to-male transmission **(Fig. 5)**.

Examples: Familial hypophosphatemic rickets, Rett syndrome, and Aicardi syndrome.

■ X-LINKED RECESSIVE

Males have a single X chromosome and are therefore hemizygous for most of the genes present on the X chromosome.

Hence, males are affected almost exclusively.

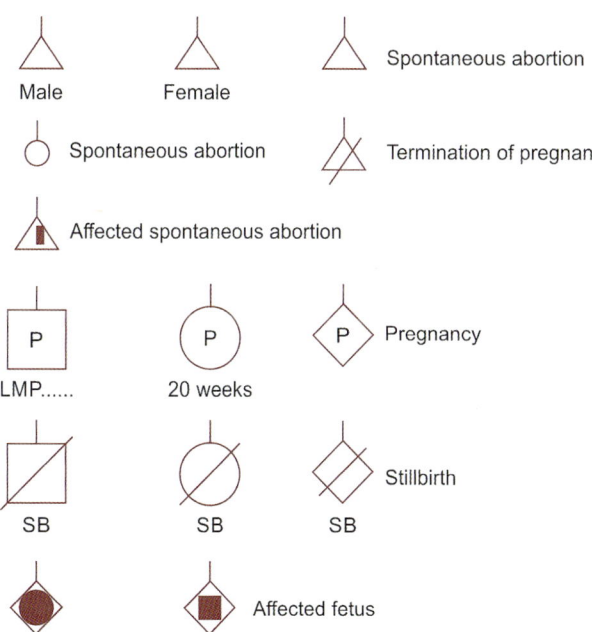

Fig. 2: Pedigree symbols for pregnancies not carried till term. (LMP: last menstrual period)

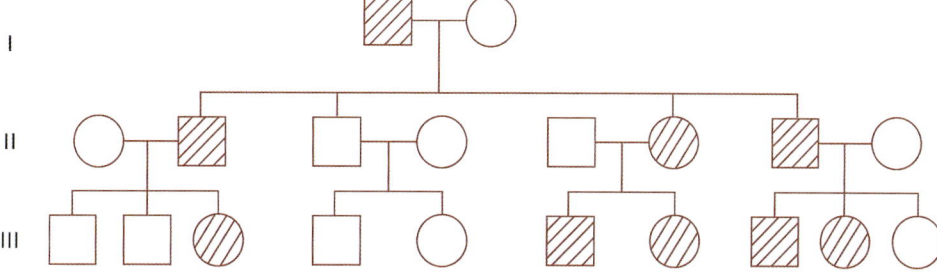

Fig. 3: Pedigree chart showing autosomal dominant inheritance.

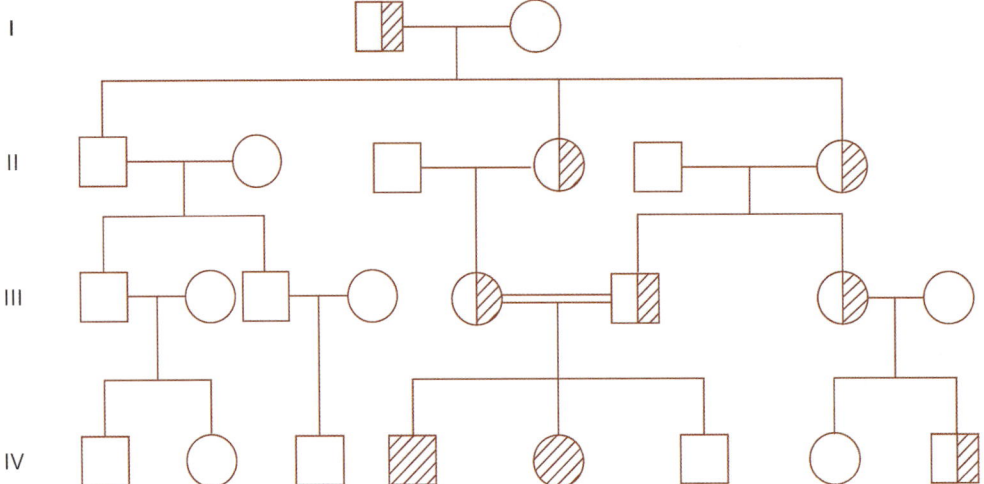

Fig. 4: Pedigree chart showing autosomal recessive disorder.

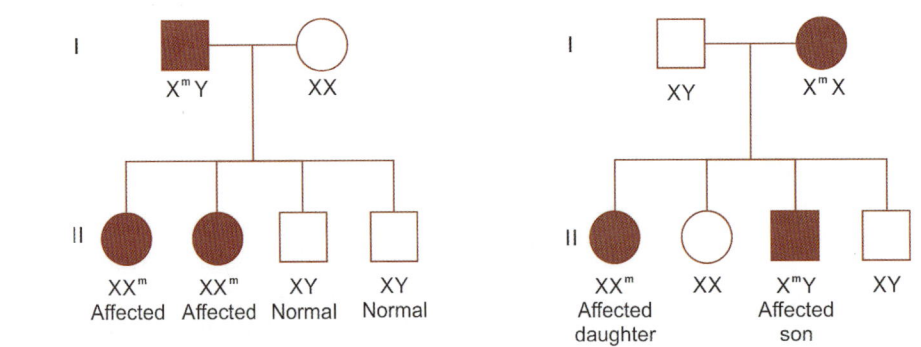

Fig. 5: Pedigree chart showing X-linked dominant inheritance.

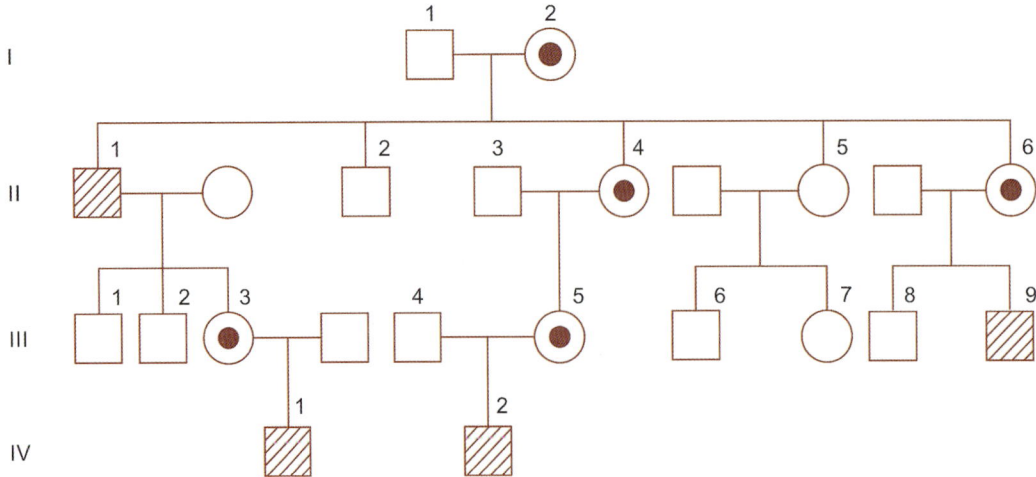

Fig. 6: Pedigree showing X-linked recessive inheritance.

No male-to-male transmission as the X chromosome in a male is contributed by the mother.

Males pass the gene to the daughters, who become carriers and may have affected sons **(Fig. 6)**.

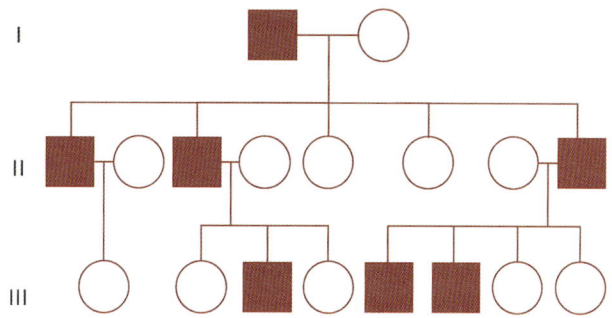

Fig. 7: Pedigree showing Y-linked inheritance.

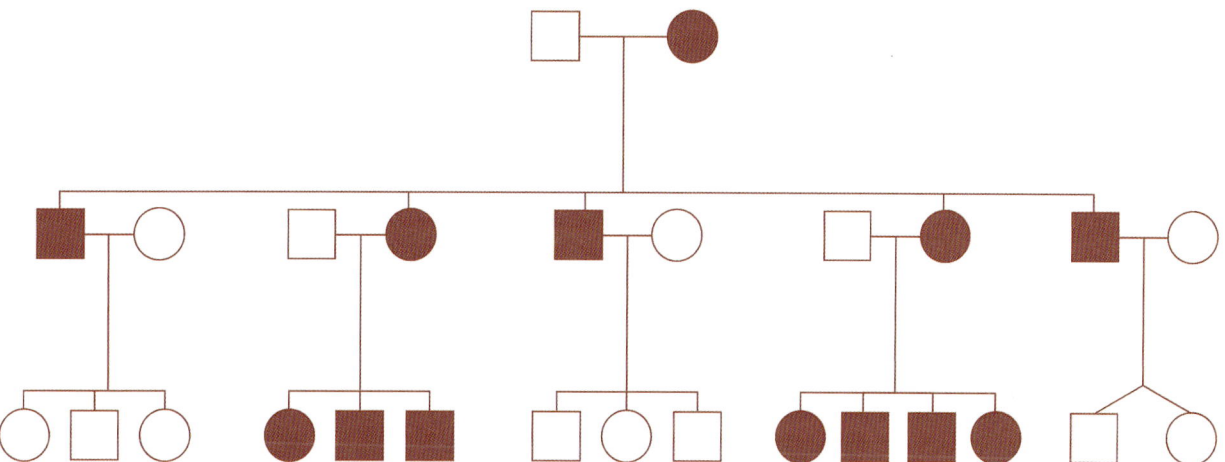

Fig. 8: Pedigree showing mitochondrial inheritance.

Examples: Duchenne muscular dystrophy, red-green color blindness, and hemophilia.

Y-LINKED DISORDERS

Rare as very few genes are located on the Y chromosome.

The trait/disorder is passed on by the fathers to the sons **(Fig. 7)**.

Example: Hypertrichosis of ears.

MITOCHONDRIAL INHERITANCE

This is a non-Mendelian inheritance. Affection of disease depends upon various factors such as heteroplasmy, homoplasmy, and bottleneck phenomena.

These traits/disorders are passed on by an affected/carrier mother to all of her offspring.

Affected fathers do not pass the trait to his children.

Both males and females may be affected **(Fig. 8)**.

Examples: Leber's hereditary optic neuropathy, mitochondrial encephalopathy, lactic acidosis, and stroke-like episodes (MELAS) syndrome.

CONCLUSION

Pedigree analysis is thus drawing inferences on the mode of transmission and probability of inheritance by collating all the information gathered like pieces of jigsaw puzzle to build a full picture. It helps to suspect or diagnose a genetic disorder in the family, predict the genetic risk and calculate risk of recurrence. It is an important and essential component of genetic history taking and counseling. Every clinician should be familiar with how to draw and interpret a basic pedigree chart.

REFERENCES

1. Phadke SR. Genetics for Clinicians. Prism Publications; 2006.
2. Adam MP, Mirzaa GM, Pagon RA, Wallace SE, Bean LJH, Grippet KW, et al. (Eds). Gene Reviews. Seattle (WA): University of Washington, Seattle; 1993-2023.
3. Kingdom R, Wright CF. Incomplete penetrance and variable expressivity: from clinical studies to population cohorts. Front Genet. 2022;13:920390.

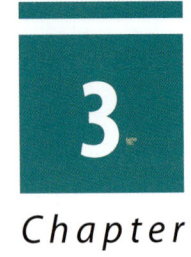

Chapter 3

Carrier Screening and Genetic Inheritance

Malathi G Prasad, Safa Abdul Syed Basheerudeen

■ GENETIC CARRIER TESTING/SCREENING

The term "carrier" in genetics is referred to the individual who has a copy of a genomic variant linked to a disease or disorder and has the potential to pass it on to the next generation. The term "screening" refers to the process of identifying asymptomatic patients within a population. Carrier screening in genetics attempts to determine, among asymptomatic patients, those capable of passing genes or genetic risk to future generations. The target populations are couples who are pregnant or planning to become pregnant. Identifying carriers of autosomal recessive (AR) or X-linked disorders early in pregnancy is beneficial to prospective parents. Couples can get related information and become aware of the probable genetic risks to their progeny and of the various available reproductive options which include, prenatal diagnosis followed by continuation or termination of pregnancy due to fetus being affected by disease or disorder and having a choice to choose preimplantation genetic diagnosis, by using donor sperm or oocytes, seeking adoption or refraining from producing children.[1]

■ GENETIC INHERITANCE PATTERN

Genetic traits are determined by the sequence of deoxyribonucleic acid (DNA) nucleotides in an organism's genome. The human genome is made up of 23 pairs of chromosomes, with one set of chromosomes, in each pair, coming from each parent. There are several different modes of genetic inheritance, including dominant, recessive, X-linked, and mitochondrial inheritance. Each of these modes of inheritance has different implications for the variability and expressivity and risk of diseases and disorders.[2]

- *Dominant inheritance:* It occurs when a single copy of a mutated gene is sufficient to cause a particular trait or disorder. In other words, if one parent has the dominant gene mutation, there is a 50% chance that their offspring will inherit the mutation and the corresponding trait or disorder.

  Examples of conditions that follow dominant inheritance include Huntington's disease and Marfan syndrome.

- *Recessive inheritance:* It occurs when two copies of a mutated gene are necessary to cause a particular trait or disorder. If both parents carry one copy of the mutated gene, there is a 25% chance that their offspring will inherit two copies of the gene and the corresponding trait or disorder. For example, beta thalassemia is inherited in AR pattern which is for a child to be born with beta thalassemia, he/she has to inherit a copy of the faulty beta thalassemia gene from both the parents.

  Examples of conditions that follow recessive inheritance include cystic fibrosis (CF), sickle cell anemia, and Tay–Sachs disease. Inborn errors of metabolic disorders are mostly inherited in AR fashion.

- *X-linked inheritance:* It refers to the inheritance of genes located on the X chromosome, which is one of the two sex chromosomes. Because males only inherit one copy of X chromosome (from their mother), X-linked traits, or disorders are often more common and severe in males, e.g., Duchenne muscular dystrophy (DMD). If a female is a carrier of an X-linked trait or disorder, there is a 50% chance that her male offspring will inherit the trait or disorder.
  - *X-linked dominant disorders:* Fragile X syndrome, Rett syndrome, the X-linked lissencephaly and double-cortex syndrome, and incontinentia pigmenti type 1.
  - *X-linked recessive disorders:* Fabry disease, red-green color blindness, nonspecific X-linked mental

retardation, Duchenne muscular dystrophy, Becker muscular dystrophy, hemophilia A (factor VIII), hemophilia B (factor IX), and X-linked ichthyosis.

- *Mitochondrial inheritance:* It refers to the inheritance of genes located in the mitochondria, which are organelles that produce energy for the cell. Mitochondrial DNA is inherited exclusively from the mother. Therefore, any mitochondrial mutations will be passed down from the mother to all of her offspring.

  Examples of conditions that follow mitochondrial inheritance include Leber's hereditary optic neuropathy and mitochondrial encephalopathy.

■ TYPES OF GENETIC TESTS

The following are some of the common types of genetic carrier screening tests:

Biochemical Tests

These tests are used to measure the levels of specific enzymes or protein markers in the blood that are produced by specific genes. If the levels of these enzymes or proteins are abnormal, it can indicate that the individual is a carrier for a specific genetic disorder. These groups of disorders caused due to congenital aberrant metabolism are called as inborn errors in metabolic (IEM) disorders. Examples of IEM's disorders include fructose intolerance, galactosemia, Maple syrup urine disease (MSUD), and phenylketonuria (PKU).

Examples of biochemical genetic tests include measuring the levels of beta-galactosidase for Tay–Sachs disease and levels of hexosaminidase A for Sandhoff disease.

Chromosome Analysis

Chromosome analysis by chromosomal microarray (CMA) or a simple karyotype is used to detect numerical and structural aneuploidies, which include loss of, or addition of extra chromosomes that can cause genetic disorders. Karyotyping also aids in examining the chromosomes for insertions, deletions, duplications, inversions, and translocations.

Examples of disorders that are studied through karyotyping—trisomy 13, 18, and 21, Robertsonian translocations, 5p deletion syndrome, Klinefelter syndrome (47XXY), Turner syndrome (45X), and Jacobs syndrome (47XYY).

Deoxyribonucleic Acid–based Tests

These tests are used to detect specific genetic mutations by analyzing the DNA sequence of a person's genes. There are two main types of DNA tests—targeted mutation analysis and sequencing. Targeted mutation analysis is used to detect a specific known mutation that is associated with a genetic disorder, while sequencing is used to analyze the entire coding region (exome) of a gene to identify any genetic mutations that may be present.

- *Next generation sequencing (NGS):* All regions of the genome that code for amino acids of an individual's genome are referred as an exome. Sequencing technology has advanced in such a way that high-throughput sequencing at low cost for an entire exome is now possible. There are four types of NGS which include automated NGS, parallel NGS, high throughput DNA NGS, and high throughput ribonucleic acid (RNA) NGS. Sequence data for an entire exome can now be obtained in <20 days. The latest addition of pan-ethnic carrier screening incorporates NGS technology or the ability to sequence across regions of the genome that include genes of interest. Screening now includes not only common recessive conditions but rare recessive conditions, semidominant (e.g., factor V Leiden) conditions, and X-linked (e.g., Fragile X mental retardation) conditions. Importantly, couples may learn they are not only asymptomatic carriers but presymptomatic carriers too. NGS is highly accurate and helps in simultaneously testing a significantly larger number of alleles from a single sample.[3]
- *Carrier testing:* The following are two types of carrier screening/testing:
  1. *Targeted carrier testing:* These specific panel tests are offered to individuals belonging to high-risk population or ethnic groups that are known to be carriers of genes for a particular disorder.

     For example, carrier testing is highly recommended to individuals belonging to Ashkenazi Jewish heritage who plan to have children or are pregnant. Diseases/disorders prevalent in individuals belonging to this ethnicity include—CF, Canavan disease, familial dysautonomia, Tay–Sachs disease, Fanconi anemia, Niemann–Pick disease, Bloom syndrome, mucolipidosis type IV, and Gaucher disease.

     Thalassemia mainly affects people who are from, or who have family members originally from—around the Mediterranean, including Italy, Greece, and Cyprus.

Sickle cell disease is commonly prevalent in population of African descent.

In India, Thalassemia is widespread across the country, but is found to be prevalent in higher frequencies among certain communities such as the Sindhis, Punjabis, Gujaratis, Bengalis, Mahars, Kolis, Saraswats, Lohanas, and Gaurs. Whereas, the highest number of cases of Sickle cell disease is seen in the tribal population of India, which includes the Bhils, Madias, Pawaras, Pardhans, and Otkars.

2. *Expanded carrier screening (ECS):* Genotyping technology available two decades ago helped in the molecular diagnosis of conditions which were characterized by a severe phenotype within families (e.g., CF). With the advancement of sequencing technology, the capability to analyze multiple genes and sequence variants within the same sample became more efficient that paved way for array of screening panels. This led to a new name called *ECS*, which allows screening of more than hundred different disorders, which are not restricted to a specific population screening. Traditional carrier screening utilized simpler technologies such as Sanger sequencing or low density microarray which were both time-consuming and cumbersome, ECS is more focused on high throughput applications which uses NGS and high density microarray technologies making it more accurate, speedy, and a go to test option to pick up subtle changes in an individual genome. In the clinical setting, ECS has extended beyond asymptomatic carriers of recessive conditions to include presymptomatic carriers of X-linked and semidominant conditions. ECS is vital in picking up severe disorders that affects individual's quality of life from an early age and is useful in identifying presymptomatic risk that helps patients and clinicians stay informed. However, for some individuals, this abundant information may lead to anxiety, stress, and trauma especially when presymptomatic and late onset disorders conditions are known beforehand. Anxiety can also originate from the identification of variants with uncertain significance (VUS), hence care must be taken by the clinician and genetic counselors to educate and counsel in a medically literate fashion. While exhaustive literature is available for CF and hemoglobinopathies (HbPs) that highlight the importance and positive approach toward mandatory global carrier screening programs, carrier testing is still usually restricted to at risk families and partners of CF patients and carriers. This may be attributed to the individual's psychological burden and risk of stigmatization by the society of being a carrier.[4-6]

THE AMERICAN COLLEGE OF OBSTETRICIANS AND GYNECOLOGISTS RECOMMENDATIONS

The American College of Obstetricians and Gynecologists (ACOG) guidance: ACOG issued a committee opinion in March 2017 regarding ECS in the age of genomic medicine, which included the following opinions.[7]

- The American College of Obstetricians and Gynecologists recommends offering pan-ethnic carrier screening for the following two conditions that is CF and spinal muscular atrophy (SMA).
- Individuals should have freedom of choice with respect to ECS.
- A complete blood count (CBC) is a general screen for anemia and is a first-line screen for some (HbPs). Hemoglobin electrophoresis is recommended for patients with African, Mediterranean, Middle Eastern, Southeast Asian, or West Indian ancestry.
- Couples with consanguinity should be offered genetic counseling for the increased risk of AR disorders.
- Individuals undergoing ECS should be counseled concerning the residual risk with any test result.
- If a carrier couple is identified before pregnancy, genetic counseling is encouraged so that reproductive options can be discussed.
- The American College of Obstetricians and Gynecologists recommends offering Ashkenazi Jews screening for Tay–Sachs and Canavan diseases as well as familial dysautonomia, due to high frequency of this disease burden present in Ashkenazi ethnicity.
- When patients/couples select screening for more conditions than those recommended by ACOG, they are selecting ECS and they may receive results for some conditions that could affect their own health. These conditions include dominant, semidominant, presymptomatic, and X-linked conditions. Proper pretest and post-test counseling is advised.

- Expanded carrier screening gene panels should not include conditions associated with a disease of adult onset. ACOG recognized that *ECS* gene panels may change over time and that there may be differences in the conditions screened.
- A follow-up publication from the ACOG, which replaced its previous reports on carrier screening, contains recommendations regarding screening for SMA, CF, HbPs, Fragile X syndrome (FXS), and genetic conditions in Ashkenazi Jewish individuals.[8]

TAKE HOME MESSAGES

- Carrier testing mainly focuses on the individuals who do have a higher a priori risk for having a child with a certain disease based on their or their partners' personal or familial history.
- If both parents are carriers for a genetic disorder that follows AR inheritance, there is a 25% chance that their child will inherit two copies of the mutated gene and develop the disorder.
- Majority of the available screening programs aims at preventing, treating, and alleviating the disease burden from the population, but the goal of preconception carrier testing by ECS is to provide information to the couple so as to support their reproductive autonomy and arrive at an informed decision making.
- Carrier testing when performed preconception; it takes away the couples emotional stress and pressures, than when a test is performed during pregnancy.

CONCLUSION

Carrier screening is beneficial, as it aids in providing information to the couple about the extent of risk, of passing on the defective gene copy to their progeny, thereby, helping the couple make informed decision and supporting their reproductive autonomy.

REFERENCES

1. Antonarakis SE. Carrier screening for recessive disorders. Nat Rev Genet. 2019;20(9):549-61.
2. Verma IC, Puri RD. Global burden of genetic disease and the role of genetic screening. Semin Fetal Neonatal Med. 2015;20(5):354-63.
3. Kraft SA, Devan D, Benjamin SW, Katrina ABG. The evolving landscape of expanded carrier screening: challenges and opportunities. Genet Med. 2019;21(4):790-7.
4. Taylor-Cousar JL, Munck A, McKone EF, Van Der Ent CK, Moeller A, Simard C, et al. Tezacaftor–ivacaftor in patients with cystic fibrosis homozygous for Phe508del. N Engl J Med. 2017;377(21):2013-23.
5. ACOG Committee Opinion No. 486: update on carrier screening for cystic fibrosis. Obstet Gynecol. 2011;117(4):1028-31.
6. Haque IS, Lazarin GA, Kang HP, Evans EA, Goldberg JD, Wapner RJ. Modeled fetal risk of genetic diseases identified by expanded carrier screening. JAMA. 2016;316(7):734-42.
7. Committee opinion no. 690 summary: carrier screening in the age of genomic medicine. Obstet Gynecol. 2017;129(3):595-6.
8. Committee opinion no. 691: carrier screening for genetic conditions. Obstet Gynecol. 2017;129(3):e41-55.

Preconception Genetic Counseling

Deepti Gupta, Dpankar Banerji

■ INTRODUCTION

With the rising incidence in genetic disorders and advancing technologies, genetic counseling is now an integral part of obstetric practice. Situation is particularly unique and relevant in India because of cultural heterogeneity of population base, varied marriage practices including consanguinity. In terms of geographical area India is sixth largest but most populous now. Indian population seems to have evolved from 4 to 5 ancestry groups owing to multiple migratory waves.[1] Prevalence of birth defects reported in India is about 64.4/1,000 births[1] **(Table 1)**. Inborn errors of metabolism, Down syndrome, hemoglobinopathies are the common disorders encountered. Diseases which affect minimal population are called rare diseases or "orphan diseases". According to the "Rare Disease Terminology and Definitions Used in Outcomes Research Working Group," any disease with global prevalence of 40–50 disease/100,000 people can be referred to as rare disease.[2] Indian Council of Medical Research (ICMR) defines, rare disease in India as one with prevalence of one in 2,500,[3] however Organization for Rare Diseases in India (ORDI) suggests threshold of one in 5,000.[4] Genetic factors are responsible for 40% of rare diseases[5] and even with small prevalence, in a populous country like India they constitute a large volume.

Since obstetrician/gynecologist is the primary care provider for most women of reproductive age group, they must be well versed with preconception genetic counseling.

■ DEFINITION

Genetic counseling is process of communication wherein trained professionals help patients understand the medical, psychosocial, familial implications of genetic contributions to disease.[6] It can also be described as a process through which individuals who are either affected by, or may be at risk of developing, a condition with a genetic basis, or are at risk of having children affected by such a condition, receive information and advice about its natural history and management, its transmission, and the available reproductive options.

Usually, it involves:
- Interpretation of family and medical histories
- Assessing chance of disease occurrence/recurrence
- Education about hereditary pattern, diagnosis, management, and prevention
- Counseling and adaptation to options

Obstetrician should remember that goal of counseling is providing balanced information to help patient make informed choice and not simply testing.[7] Preconception counseling and care primarily aims to educate individuals and couples, assess risks, optimize medical care, and offer interventions before pregnancy to minimize the likelihood of poor pregnancy-related outcomes.

■ RISK ASSESSMENT

This is an important and first component of successful genetic counseling. Proper risk assessment also allows

TABLE 1: List of genetic disease with estimated prevalence.[1]

Disease	Frequency	State/region
Hemophilia A	0.9/100,000	Across India
Hemophilia B	0.1/100,000	Across India
Sickle cell anemia	2–20%	Across India
Beta thalassemia trait	3–4%	Across India
Duchenne muscular dystrophy and spinal muscular atrophy	1 in 1,400 male live births	Southern India
Skeletal dysplasia	19.6/10,000 newborns	Southern India

> **BOX 1:** Family history red flags to prompt further genetic counseling.[6]
>
> *Red flags in family history:*
> - Known or suspected genetic condition in family
> - Ethnic predisposition to certain genetic disorders
> - Consanguinity
> - Earlier than expected onset of disease
> - One or more major malformation
> - Growth abnormalities
> - Intellectual disability or developmental delay
> - Recurrent pregnancy loss >2

> **BOX 2:** Things to remember while choosing genetic laboratory.
>
> *Things to remember:*
> - Test performance—sensitivity, specificity, positive predictive value, negative predictive value, and test failure rate
> - Test logistics—sample to be procured, transportation requirements, and turnaround time
> - Test reporting—parameters included, clarity of results, and communication of abnormal results
> - Support provided—genetic expert availability if needed and genetic counseling services available if needed
> - Billing—liaison with insurance plans and payment plan options

for correct test selection and interpretation. Risk assessment includes thorough age, ethnicity, medical, family history, pregnancy, exposure, and travel histories, history of consanguinity. Regular practice of detailed family history helps in identifying increased risks of inherited conditions, birth defects, hereditary cancers, and medical conditions with genetic predisposition like diabetes **(Box 1)**.

Three generation pedigree chart or patient questionnaire may be employed to elicit details.

■ GENETIC TESTING

Genetic testing can be either part of routine prenatal care or based on specific risk factor identified. There is a gamut of test available and identification of appropriate facility and test is empirical for cost-effective prenatal testing. Wherever needed or appropriate, advice of clinical geneticist must be solicited. We now have an entire spectrum of screening options including preconception carrier screening (PCS), extended preconception carrier screening (ECS), preimplantation genetic testing for aneuploidy (PGT-A) [previously referred to as preimplantation genetic screening (PGS)], preimplantation genetic testing for monogenic effects (PGT-M) [previously referred to as preimplantation genetic diagnosis (PGD)].[8] Some learn about carrier status through routine PCS while others are subjected to specific PGT-M based on previously affected child/family history.

The concept at center of PCS is thought to be increasing reproductive autonomy of couples and providing them knowledge about available treatment options[8] **(Box 2)**.

> **BOX 3:** Components of pretest counseling.
>
> - Purpose of the test
> - Test procedure
> - Test accuracy, etc.
> - Risks of testing—complications, uncertain results, and incidental findings
> - Benefits of testing
> - Possible results—implications and management options
> - Turnaround time and payment options
> - Result communication

■ PRETEST COUNSELING

This is perhaps one of the most important components of entire prenatal counseling. Balanced information about justification of test, alternative testing options if any, expected results/outcomes and management options/what to expect with continuation of pregnancy in case of positive test result must be given. The idea should be to facilitate autonomous decision. The topics of discussion need to be individualized based on suspected anomaly and test being ordered. For example, PGT-A would focus more on aneuploidy rates and mosaicism. Another important fact to consider is the chronological age at time of testing. Embryos show far higher rates of aneuploidy than viable intrauterine pregnancies, and rates further drop as pregnancies advance.[8] During pretest counseling, variants not screened due to technical limitations, harmful mutations not yet identified, gonadal mosaicism, and de novo mutations should be kept in mind **(Box 3)**.

Every session must be thoroughly documented even if the patient declines genetic testing. Pretest counseling should ideally be nondirective in nature, in accordance with patient's culture, education, language, and values.

Different counseling aids such as videos, tutorials, and pictorial charts may be used. A lot of these tests are very expensive and not freely available in government facilities; hence insurance coverage should be checked too.

■ POST-TEST COUNSELING

Any test result could potentially imply that couple has a good chance of having an affected baby. The couple could then accept the risk, choose to not have a child, pursue adoption, opt gamete donation, or prefer PGT-M of embryos formed though in vitro fertilization (IVF).[9] Post-test counseling should be planned keeping in mind previous history. Some couples may have affected child/family history and would be more mentally prepared for confirmation of diagnosis, for others the results may come as a complete unanticipated surprise. Another important feature to remember is "penetrance" as all genetic conditions do not have 100% penetrance. In simple terms it means with positive result, parents are confronted with odds of different diseases child might develop or might not. This concern could lead to termination of otherwise healthy pregnancies, a phenomenon described as "healthy ill." Thus, largely post-test counseling would involve discussion about pregnancy termination in case of positive result or preparing for birth of child with special needs (physical and/or emotional).

■ CONCLUSION

Preconception screening fills a potential gap in reproductive medicines, because most individuals testing positive as carrier will not have a positive family history for that disorder. With widespread test availability, decreasing costs, and increasing incidences, clinicians should consider "universal screening" to ensure reproductive justice and identify subclinical carriers. Any genetic testing should be elective and not a mandatory medical test.

■ REFERENCES

1. The GUaRDIAN Consortium; Sivasubbu S, Scaria V. Genomics of rare genetic diseases—experiences from India. Hum Genomics. 2019;14(1):52.
2. Richter T, Nestler-Parr S, Babela R, Khan ZM, Tesoro T, Molsen E, et al. Rare disease terminology and definitions—a systematic global review: report of the ISPOR Rare Disease Special Interest Group. Value Health. 2015;18(6):906-14.
3. Swaminathan S. (2017). ICMR Bulletin. [online] Available from: https://www.icmr.nic.in/sites/default/files/icmr_bulletins/Apr_Jun_2017.pdf [Last accessed October, 2023].
4. Rajasimha HK, Shirol PB, Ramamoorthy P, Hegde M, Barde S, Chandru V, et al. Organization for rare diseases India (ORDI)—addressing the challenges and opportunities for the Indian rare diseases' community. Genet Res (Camb). 2014;96:e009.
5. Ferreira CR. The burden of rare diseases. Am J Med Genet A. 2019;179(6):885-92.
6. Hoskovec Jennifer M, Stevens Blair K. Genetic Counseling-overview for the obstetrician gynecologist. Obstet Gynecol Clin North Am. 2018;45(1):1-12.
7. Ioannides AS. Preconception and prenatal genetic counselling. Best Pract Res Clin Obstet Gynaecol. 2017;42:2-10.
8. Black DL, Fischer JM. Genetic counseling for pre-implantation genetic testing. In: Griffin DK, Harton GL (Eds). Preimplantation Genetic Testing Recent Advances in Reproductive Medicine. 1st edition. CRC Press; 2020.
9. Greenfield DA. Psychological aspects of reproductive genetic screening and diagnoses. In: Garcia-Velasco JA, Seli E. Human Reproductive Genetics. 1st edition. Academic Press Publication; 2020.

Chapter 5: Genetic Tests and their Significance in Prenatal Evaluation

Shyama Devadasan

INTRODUCTION

Advances in scientific research and technology have revolutionized the field of prenatal evaluation, offering expectant parents a deeper understanding of their unborn child's genetic makeup. Genetic tests have become a vital tool in prenatal care, providing valuable insights into potential health risks, inherited disorders, and chromosomal abnormalities. This chapter explores the theoretical significance of genetic tests in prenatal evaluation, shedding light on their role in enhancing our understanding of human development and promoting informed decision-making. The results of these tests help parents and healthcare professionals make informed decisions about the pregnancy, including the management of any potential health concerns.

NONINVASIVE PRENATAL SCREENING

One of the most common and recent genetic tests conducted during prenatal evaluation is the noninvasive prenatal screening (NIPS) or cell-free DNA (cfDNA) test[1] **(Table 1)**. This test involves analyzing a small sample of the mother's blood to detect fragments of the fetus's DNA. It has a detection rate of up to 99% for the common aneuploidies (trisomy 21, 18, and 13) with false positive rates as low as 0.1%. NIPS has a lower risk of complications compared to invasive procedures[2] such as amniocentesis or chorionic villus sampling (CVS). But, nevertheless it is a screening test and any abnormality has to be confirmed with a definitive diagnostic testing. Apart from this, the use of NIPS for identification of other rare trisomies or microdeletions/duplications is not yet recommended for routine use and is currently under investigation.

DIAGNOSTIC PROCEDURES

All prenatal diagnostic tests[3] require an invasive procedure to obtain the sample for analysis. These procedures include

TABLE 1: Cell-free DNA detection and false positive rates for common aneuploidy.

Condition	Detection rate (%)	False positive rate (%)
Trisomy 21	99.7 (99.1–99.9)	0.04 (0.02–0.07)
Trisomy 18	97.9 (94.9–99.1)	0.04 (0.03–0.07)
Trisomy 13	99.0 (65.8–100)	0.04 (0.02–0.07)
Monosomy X	95.8 (70.3–99.5)	0.14 (0.06–0.38)
Sex chromosome aneuploidy[a]	100 (83–100)	0.004 (0.0–0.08)

[a]Including XXX, XXY, and XYY
Source: Adapted from Gil MM, Brik M, Casanova C, Martin-Alonso R, Verdejo M, Ramírez E, et al. Screening for trisomies 21 and 18 in a Spanish public hospital: from the combined test to the cell-free DNA test. J Matern Fetal Neonatal Med. 2017;30(20):2476-82.

CVS, amniocentesis, and less commonly performed fetal blood sampling (FBS). These invasive procedures carry a risk of fetal loss (rate of 0.5%) compared to NIPS but offer more comprehensive genetic information **(Table 2)**.

Chorionic Villus Sampling

Chorionic villus sampling is performed between 11 and 14 weeks of gestation by transabdominal or transcervical route according to operator's experience or placental location using 18–20G needle under continuous ultrasound guidance **(Fig. 1)**. This procedure involves aspiration of minimum 5–10 mg of villi (trophoblastic cells) from the placenta. Chorionic tissue has ample amount of DNA material and is especially useful for DNA-based tests. In addition, cytogenetic study from chorionic tissue culture takes less turnaround time.

It is recommended not to perform CVS before 10 completed weeks of gestation, due to higher risk of fetal loss and complications such as limb reduction defects/oromandibular hypoplasia reported in literature. This is because the limbs and mandible are more susceptible to vascular disruption before 10 weeks.

TABLE 2: Diagnostic procedures and types of available tests.			
Procedure	Sample	Timing	Tests
CVS	Chorionic villi	11–14 weeks	Karyotype, microarray, DNA testing
Amniocentesis	Amniotic fluid	16 weeks onward	Karyotype, microarray, DNA testing, enzyme testing, fetal AFP, viral PCR
FBS	Fetal blood	18 weeks onward	Karyotype, microarray, DNA testing, fetal AFP, viral PCR

(AFP: alpha-fetoprotein; CVS: chorionic villus sampling; DNA: deoxyribonucleic acid; FBS: fetal blood sampling; PCR: polymerase chain reaction)

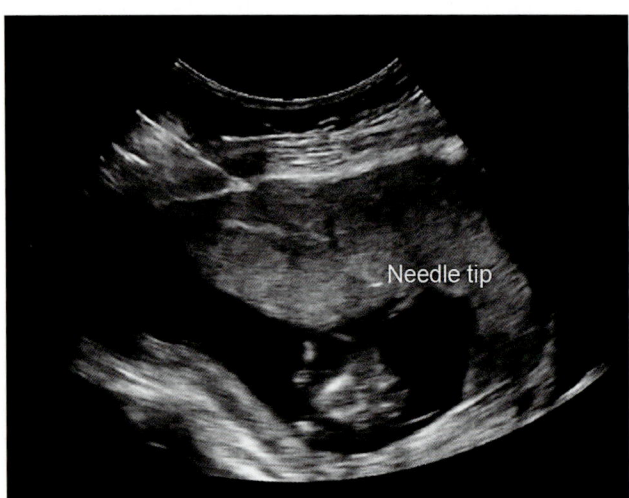

Fig. 1: Ultrasound scan image during chorionic villus sampling.

Complications include fetal loss (0.2–2%), vaginal bleeding (10%), amniotic fluid leakage (<0.5%), and chorioamnionitis (1–2 in 3,000). Fetal loss rates are slightly higher with transcervical route as compared to transabdominal route and increase with number of needle insertion and gestational age <10 weeks. Presence of fetal structural malformation or an increased nuchal translucency or a low pregnancy-associated plasma protein-A (PAPP-A) in the maternal serum screen are associated with a background increased risk of miscarriage even before a CVS. Risk of miscarriage decreases obviously with better operator experience.

Failure of trophoblast culture may be seen in 0.5% of samples. Placental mosaicism is seen in 1% of CVS cultures. Hence, in few such cases a repeat invasive procedure of amniocentesis or cordocentesis may be required to differentiate true fetal mosaicism from confined placental mosaicism.

Benefit of CVS over amniocentesis is an early diagnosis so that informed decisions about pregnancy can be taken by the couple earlier.

Amniocentesis

Amniocentesis involves the transabdominal aspiration of amniotic fluid (around 15–30 mL) from the uterine cavity using 20–22G spinal needle under continuous ultrasound guidance. The amniotic fluid containing fetal cells is then analyzed for fetal karyotype to detect chromosomal abnormalities as well as other genetic disorders, alpha-fetoprotein level or acetylcholine level for open neural tube defects **(Figs. 2A and B)**.

It is recommended to perform amniocentesis at or beyond 15^{+0} completed weeks of gestation as higher rate of total fetal losses, fetal talipes and postprocedure amniotic fluid leakage have been reported in cases of early amniocentesis done prior to 14 weeks.

Complications include risk of fetal loss varying from 0.1 to 1%, postprocedure membrane rupture in 1–2%, chorioamnionitis (<0.1%), needle injury to the fetus and maternal sepsis in very rare circumstances. However, in women with iatrogenic leak following amniocentesis, spontaneous sealing of the membranes is commonly seen.

Lower fetal loss rates have been documented with better operator experience of >100 procedures per annum. If more than two punctures have been attempted, it is ideal that the procedure be postponed by 24 hours. Use of 20G or 22G needle is associated with similar loss rates. The presence of fetal structural anomalies itself places the pregnancy at higher background risk of miscarriage and the risk increases further following amniocentesis. A bloody or brown discolored tap reflects intraamniotic bleeding and is associated with a higher postprocedure fetal loss.

Failure of amniocytes to culture is reported in 0.1% of procedures and is more with advanced gestational age at amniocentesis and a blood stained tap.

Fetal Blood Sampling

Cordocentesis involves ultrasound-guided puncture of umbilical cord (umbilical vein), using 20–22G needle

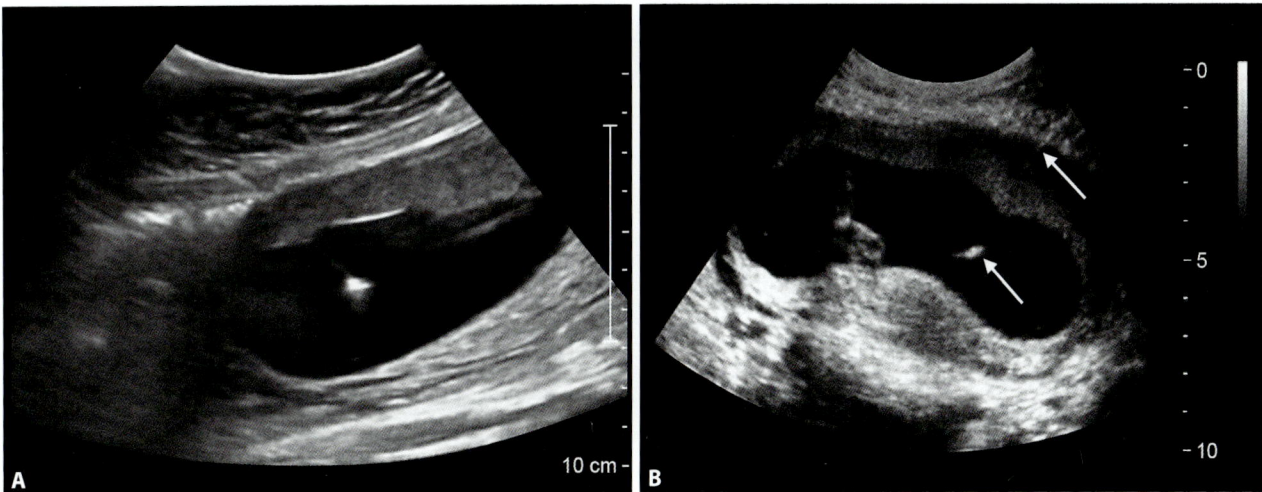

Figs. 2A and B: Ultrasound scan image during amniocentesis.

under continuous ultrasound guidance for either diagnostic (FBS) or therapeutic (intrauterine transfusion or drug instillation) purposes. It is performed beyond 18^{+0} completed weeks of gestation (due to increased fetal loss rate if performed earlier). Fetal blood can be sampled either from the placental cord insertion site, fetal intrahepatic portal vein, or a free loop of cord.

It is usually associated with 1–2% risk of fetal loss. Complications include amniotic fluid leak, chorioamnionitis, cord hematoma, transient bradycardia, bleeding from the needle site, fetomaternal hemorrhage, and rarely fetal demise. Increased risk of fetal loss may be associated with fetal anomalies, hydrops, fetal growth restriction, and gestational age of <24 weeks at sampling.

This direct sampling is less commonly used, as the above modalities of fetal cells sampling are technically easier and safer. Specific indications for FBS are:
- Fetal blood sampling is especially indicated in fetus at higher risk for hematological disorders such as hemophilia and hemoglobinopathy.
- Identify genetic disorders where amniocentesis or CVS are inconclusive or unsuccessful like placental mosaicism.
- Suspected fetal anemia-Rh sensitized, parvo virus, chronic fetomaternal hemorrhage, hydrops (quantification of fetal anemia or platelet/lymphocyte count)
- Alloimmune thrombocytopenia
- Along with intrauterine transfusion in Rh isoimmunized
- Along with therapeutic procedures—arrhythmias, fetal thyroid disease
- No amniotic fluid is available for sampling (anhydramnios).

INDICATIONS OF PRENATAL GENETIC TESTING[4,5]

These tests can be performed at different stages of pregnancy and are typically recommended for individuals with certain risk factors.
- High risk aneuploidy screening test results from first trimester combined screening/NIPS/second trimester triple or quadruple test.
- A previous pregnancy that resulted in a fetus or an infant with chromosome abnormalities.
- One parent with a balanced chromosome translocation.
- A family history of known genetic disorder like metabolic disease for which the enzyme defect is known.
- Maternal history of an X-linked disorder.
- Abnormal ultrasound examination associated with aneuploidies.
- Couples carrier for an autosomal recessive disorder, e.g., thalassemias, inborn errors of metabolism.

TYPES OF GENETIC TESTS

Genetic tests during prenatal evaluation involve analyzing the DNA or chromosomes of the fetus from the fetal sample to detect any anomalies or genetic variations. The type of testing performed on the fetal cells depends on the indication for the procedure.

Karyotype

Karyotype is the standard test to assess chromosomal abnormalities of the 23 pairs of chromosomes including sex chromosomes. The cultured fetal cells obtained from invasive tests such as CVS or amniocentesis are studied and results of karyotype are obtained in 2–3 weeks.

A karyotype can detect fetal aneuploidy[6] like a trisomy (presence of an extra chromosome such as trisomy 21), monosomy (an absence of a chromosome such as monosomy X), large deletions and duplications (large areas of extra or missing pieces of chromosome), translocations (pieces of chromosomes that have switched places), inversions, or marker and ring chromosomes. Some of these chromosomal abnormalities can be incidental findings and will not cause any phenotypic variations, while many may cause considerable disease.

Karyotype can also show mosaicism (i.e., two distinctly different cell lines present in the same sample). Mosaicism is detected in approximately 1–2% of CVS samples. The vast majority of mosaicism detected on CVS is confined to the placenta, hence referred to as confined placental mosaicism.

Chromosomal Microarray

Over the last decade, chromosomal microarray (CMA) is an important tool that provides clinically relevant information in the genetic evaluation of the fetus. It is a molecular cytogenetic technique to visualize chromosomes at a very high resolution. Other than chromosomal aneuploidies, CMA can detect smaller microdeletions/microduplications (losses or gains), which cannot be seen by a standard karyotype, such as 22q11.2 deletion syndrome (DiGeorge syndrome). These are referred to as copy number variants (CNVs). Pathogenic CNVs occur in 6% of cases with a fetal structural malformation and in 2% of structurally normal pregnancies; a much higher frequency than the 1:800 risk of Down syndrome. Hence, this is a better test when a fetal ultrasound abnormality is detected.

Some CNVs are benign and not known to cause disease. One limitation of CMA is that it can detect certain CNVs of unknown significance in around 1% of cases, also referred to as variants of unknown significance (VOUS). This can lead to a clinical dilemma and parental anxiety. Additionally, some pathogenic CNVs, such as DiGeorge syndrome, can have variable phenotypic spectrum with findings ranging from normal to mild-to-severe congenital abnormalities with or without intellectual disability. Hence, CMA needs good supportive counseling facilities by genetic counselors.

The advantage over conventional karyotyping is that CMA has a faster turnaround time of usually 15 days as it is performed on uncultured cells. However, balanced chromosome translocations are detected by karyotype only. Balanced chromosome translocations, however, are not expected to lead to a clinical phenotype, unless the breakpoint occurs in the middle of a gene. Also, CMA cannot detect single-gene disorders that cause autosomal recessive, dominant, or X-linked conditions. This requires molecular testing done either via a targeted mutation analysis or sequencing of the DNA.

Targeted Mutation Testing

Targeted gene mutation testing is usually performed only after the mutation in specific gene is known. Hence, this is useful after a carrier screening in the couple or family. For example, in sickle cell disease, when a couple is found to be carriers, fetal DNA is tested for the specific mutations carried by the parents and the diagnosis is obtained prenatally.

Additionally, targeted testing can be performed as part of familial mutation testing when a specific mutation is already known in the family and pregnancy is at risk of inheriting that condition. For example, if the father of the pregnancy has neurofibromatosis (NF) and the pathogenic mutation in the *NF1* gene is known, then the pregnancy can also be tested for the presence of that specific mutation. Expanded carrier screening panels are also available clinically.

Whole Exome Sequencing

Despite the increasing yield with CMA, almost two-thirds of fetal anomalies will not have a genetic etiology identified. It is believed that the use of whole exome sequencing (WES) prenatally will help diagnose an additional 10–30% of the remaining cases. WES can detect the mutations in protein-coding exons of over 20,000 genes, which make up to 1–2% of the genome cause >85% of all disease-causing mutations using next-generation sequencing (NGS) panels in which multiple genes are analyzed in parallel. Variants detected on WES are generally classified as in that on CMA [pathogenic, likely pathogenic, benign (not disease causing), likely benign, and VOUS]. Sequencing of the whole genome is referred to as whole genome sequencing (WGS).

Limitations of WES include longer turnaround times, high cost and detection of secondary findings in genes not associated with the fetal phenotype that may presymptomatically identify a predisposition to cancer or cardiac disease. A major challenge with new technologies such as WES and CMA is the detection of VOUS which is difficult to interpret in a prenatal setting. Variable expressivity of fetal disorders, incomplete penetrance, and presentation of ultrasound abnormalities only at late gestational ages can further complicate interpretation. Interpretation of a VOUS is highly dependent on the phenotypic information, which is often incomplete, or in some situation incorrect, due to limitations of prenatal imaging. Some phenotypes, such as intellectual disability or seizures, are simply impossible to detect on prenatal ultrasound.

Current guidelines state that prenatal exome sequencing may be considered in certain indications, either in fetuses with multiple anomalies[7] as in skeletal dysplasia or in cases of recurrent fetal abnormalities with no diagnosis by standard genetic testing. However, appropriate and thorough pretest and posttest counseling is warranted.

CONCLUSION

Genetic tests provide essential information about the genetic makeup of the fetus, enabling parents to make informed decisions and plan for the future. While the benefits of genetic testing are substantial, ethical considerations must be prioritized to ensure that individuals and families are supported and protected throughout the process. It is important to understand that many fetal anomalies may be due to multifactorial inheritance (combination of both genetic and environmental factors), epigenetic causes, or teratogenic exposures and not genetic causes alone. Also, it is essential to know that there is no test currently available that can rule out all genetic conditions and guarantee a healthy baby.[8]

REFERENCES

1. Gil MM, Brik M, Casanova C, Martin-Alonso R, Verdejo M, Ramírez E, et al. Screening for trisomies 21 and 18 in a Spanish public hospital: from the combined test to the cell-free DNA test. J Matern Fetal Neonatal Med. 2017;30(20):2476-82.
2. Ghi T, Sotiriadis A, Calda P, Costa FD, Raine-Fenning N, Alfirevic Z, et al. ISUOG Practice Guidelines: invasive procedures for prenatal diagnosis. Ultrasound Obstet Gynecol. 2016;48(2):256-68.
3. Best S, Wou K, Vora N, Van der Veyver IB, Wapner R, Chitty LS. Promises, pitfalls and practicalities of prenatal whole exome sequencing. Prenat Diagn. 2018;38(1):10-9.
4. Wou K, Chung WK, Wapner RJ. Laboratory considerations for prenatal genetic testing. Semin Perinatol. 2018;42(5): 307-13.
5. Krstić N, Običan SG. Current landscape of prenatal genetic screening and testing. Birth Defects Res. 2020;112(4):321-31.
6. Rink BD, Norton ME. Screening for fetal aneuploidy. Semin Perinatol. 2016;40(1):35-43.
7. Mone F, Quinlan-Jones E, Kilby MD. Clinical utility of exome sequencing in the prenatal diagnosis of congenital anomalies: a review. Eur J Obstet Gynecol Reprod Biol. 2018;231:19-24.
8. Phadke SR, Puri RD, Ranganath P. Prenatal screening for genetic disorders: suggested guidelines for the Indian Scenario. Indian J Med Res. 2017;146(6):689-99.

Chapter 6: Genetic Counseling in Cases of Abnormal Serum Screening

Suma Vishnu

INTRODUCTION

Prenatal testing is the best way for reducing the huge burden of genetic disorders and congenital anomalies that cause significant postnatal functional and structural impairment. Universal prenatal screening is advisable for common genetic diseases and congenital anomalies such as Down syndrome, sickle cell anemia, and neural tube defects (NTDs).

If the fetus is affected with a major genetic syndrome or congenital disorder with a poor prognosis, discontinuation of the pregnancy is an accepted strategy for reducing the burden of genetic disorders. After the birth of an affected child or an informative family history, at risk families are identified and offered appropriate genetic counseling with the option of prenatal diagnosis including invasive testing and blood tests for the condition under consideration. However, many genetic disorders and disabilities occur in families without any history of an affected child or individual. Screening tests have become available for the prevention of common genetic disorders and are being offered to all pregnant women with the advance in medical science. The disorders with a significant prevalence in India for which population-based prevention programs are needed include beta-thalassemia, sickle cell anemia, Down syndrome, and NTDs.[1-4] Prenatal diagnostic tests for these disorders should be made available through the public and private sectors in India, and awareness amongst obstetricians and primary care physicians is increasing.

The earliest noninvasive biochemical method of obtaining information about a fetus is maternal serum screening. A small group of patients that is at a sufficiently increased risk of having a fetus with a disorder is to be identified from among the healthy population. This is the objective of this test and they are to be offered a specific diagnostic test. Biochemical serum markers are used to select the women during pregnancy who may be offered amniocentesis, noninvasive prenatal testing, and other obstetric interventions. Maternal serum screen programs have the potential to decrease fetal morbidity and mortality by providing access to earlier diagnosis, by enabling families to make more informed reproductive decisions and by deciding appropriate delivery strategies.

SERUM SCREENING

The first prenatal screening test was introduced in the 1970s—a single second-trimester serum test for maternal serum alpha-fetoprotein which was a marker of NTDs. Aneuploidy screening using maternal serum markers was introduced in the 1980s, and the number and complexity of offered screening tests have been on an upward trajectory ever since. Today, we can divide prenatal genetic screening tests into four categories—(1) ultrasonography, (2) maternal carrier status of specific genetic disorders, (3) maternal serum assays which look for specific biochemical markers indicative of aneuploidy, and (4) most recently, maternal plasma fetal cell-free fetal DNA (cffDNA), which has been used for aneuploidy, microdeletion, and copy number variants (CNVs). There are four maternal serum assays which include first-trimester screening, the triple screen, the quadruple screen, and the penta screen. The option of combining first-trimester and second-trimester screening with either integrated, sequential, or contingent screening protocol can be given to the patient which provides a higher detection rate than a one-step screening.

Measurement of maternal serum levels of maternal serum alpha-fetoprotein (MSAFP), pregnancy-associated plasma protein-A (PAPP-A), free beta-human chorionic gonadotropin (beta-hCG), inhibin alpha (InhA), and unconjugated estriol is taken. cffDNA is isolated and purified from maternal plasma. The following factors can be taken into account for choosing the screening test. The mother's desire for prenatal information, family history, previous pregnancies, gestational age at the first visit, cost, and desire to pursue follow-up pregnancy care or termination in the case of an abnormal diagnostic test.

■ TYPES OF SCREENING TESTS

The earliest genetic screen is carrier screening, which ideally would be done preconception, can be done prenatally also.

Combined test: The combined test is performed in the late first trimester and includes:
- Sonographic determination of fetal nuchal translucency (NT) measured at 11^{+0} to 13^{+6} weeks
- Pregnancy associated plasma protein A (PAPP-A)
- Total/intact hCG or free hCG
- Blood for the serum markers can be drawn between 10^{+3} and 13^{+6} weeks.

Multiple marker serum-only test: A first-trimester multiple serum marker test without NT also exists, and consists of four or five of the following markers: PAPP-A, free beta hCG, InhA, placental growth factor (PlGF), and AFP, but data on performance and use are limited.

■ SECOND TRIMESTER

Quadruple marker test: The quadruple test is performed in the early second trimester optimally at 15^{+0} to 18^{+6} weeks of gestation till 22^{+6} weeks.

The most common combination includes measurement of four markers:
1. Alpha-fetoprotein
2. Unconjugated estriol (uE3)
3. Total/intact human chorionic gonadotropin (hCG) or the free beta subunit of hCG (free beta hCG)
4. Inhibin A (InhA)

A screening test utilizing cell-free DNA (cfDNA) in maternal blood is also another option for screening and has become more common over time. The methods used and the disorders that can be identified very widely. All screen for the common autosomal trisomies (13, 18, 21). Many also offer screening for fetal sex and sex chromosome abnormalities such as 45X, 47XXY, 47XYY, and 47XXX. Some whole-genome methods screen for rare autosomal trisomies such as trisomy 16. Some cfDNA tests have the option of screening for specific and larger microdeletions such as 22q11.2, 1p36 deletions and microdeletions responsible for Prader–Willi, Cri-du-chat, and Angelman syndromes. As the screening targets expand, the false-positive rate will increase and the positive-predictive values will tend to decrease due to the low prevalence of these conditions.

■ COUNSELING

Pretest counseling is a must before embarking onto any genetic screening test. Emphasis should be given on the fact that the aim of prenatal screening is limited to the identification from among apparently healthy pregnancies those at high enough risk of a given outcome to warrant the next step. It is widely recognized that for any genetic test be it screening or diagnostic, optimal pretest and post-test counseling should be offered.[5] This is particularly true for pregnant women as suboptimal pretest counseling may lead to unnecessary screening tests, anxiety and in extreme situations, ill-informed decisions for termination of pregnancy (TOP).
- A positive screening test result for aneuploidy implies that the fetus is at higher risk of having the disorder compared with the general population. It does not mean that the fetus definitely has the disorder.
- A negative result implies that your fetus is at lower risk of having the disorder compared with the general population. It does not rule out the possibility that your fetus has the disorder.

With any type of testing, there is a possibility of false-positive results and false-negative results.

■ INTERPRETATION OF RESULTS

Serum markers change with different genetic syndromes.

Levels of uE3 and AFP are, on average, lower by 30–35% [0.70–0.75 multiples of the median (MoM)] in Down syndrome pregnancies. Median PAPP-A in Down syndrome pregnancies rises from approximately 0.4 MoM at 10 weeks to approximately 0.7 MoM at 13 weeks. The first-trimester marker pattern of trisomy 18 is very low PAPP-A (median 0.1–0.2 MoM), very low free beta hCG and total/intact hCG (median 0.2–0.4 MoM) and increased NT (median 1.8–3.7 MoM). 87% of trisomy 13 cases could be detected in the first trimester with a 0.2% false-positive rate.

Prenatal serum screening results are evaluated using a patient-specific risk-based assessment. An individual's a priori risk or baseline risk is calculated based on their chronological age at the estimated date of delivery and history of a previous Down syndrome-affected pregnancy. This baseline risk is then modified by the "likelihood ratio" (LR). The LR is determined by comparing each of these serum marker MoM values with the reference values after accounting for the degree of independence between each pair of markers (measured as an R value after log transformation of the marker MoMs). The final reported risk is their calculated patient-specific risk of having a fetus affected by Down syndrome in that particular pregnancy. The goal is to optimize between higher detection rates and lower false-positive rates. The overall test performance also depends on the prevalence of the disorder in the population being screened.

Screen-positive biochemical marker-based tests: Patients who are screen positive on a biochemical marker-based test can undergo secondary screening or a diagnostic procedure. A secondary screening test aims to collect additional information about risk that screen-positive patients can have and decide whether to proceed to diagnostic testing or forgo further testing as the additional information of the secondary test has greatly reduced the risk reported by the initial screening test.

Secondary screening is best performed with cfDNA test. Because of the high sensitivity and very low false-positive rate of this test many patients with false-positive biochemical marker tests will be reclassified as screen-negative with minimal risk of misclassification as true positives. Patients who are secondary screen-positive with cfDNA should be offered an invasive test for definitive diagnosis because false-positive results are still possible (<0.1%).[6]

Alternatively, a patient who screens positive on a biochemical marker-based test may decide whether they want a definitive diagnosis, which can be provided by invasive testing [chorionic villus sampling (CVS) or amniocentesis] and a karyotype or chromosomal microarray analysis (CMA). Each approach has its own advantages and disadvantages. After a positive screening test, it is helpful for parents to meet with a genetic counselor and obstetrician to inform them of their diagnostic and management options and answer their questions.

Biochemical marker screening tests should never be repeated.[7] Repeat testing of the entire population would result in just a small increase in detection rates but is not at all justified because of the expense and risk of false reassurance or dilemmas. Repeat biochemical marker testing limited to only screen-positive patients can at times reduce the false-positive rate, but a small percentage of affected pregnancies will be incorrectly reclassified as screen-negative. However, it is important to double-check the laboratory form to make sure the patient's age, weight, gestational age, in vitro fertilization (IVF) conception, twin pregnancy, family history, etc., were recorded correctly, as these can affect the risk calculation. If an ultrasound examination has not been done, it should be performed to confirm gestational age and exclude other causes of a screen-positive test (e.g., multiple gestation, some congenital anomalies, and single fetal demise).

Screen-positive cell-free DNA-based test: Patients who opt for cfDNA screening as their initial screening test should be offered invasive testing for definitive diagnosis. In general obstetric populations, the reported positive predictive value of a positive cfDNA test result for Down syndrome ranged from 46 to 81% in three studies.[8-10] False positives can occur due to factors such as confined placental mosaicism, single fetal demise in twin pregnancy, large maternal copy-number variants, or malignancy of mother.

■ DIAGNOSTIC TESTING

Chorionic villus sampling is the best preferred diagnostic test in the first trimester and a conventional karyotype is generally obtained. Preliminary results can be available within 2 days if a direct preparation is performed and final results from cultured cells will take 7–10 days. If the cfDNA result suggests the possibility of a confined placental mosaicism, CVS will not be the preferred option. In the second trimester, amniocentesis is the best preferred option and it is performed to obtain fetal cells (amniocytes) and a conventional karyotype analysis is generally obtained. A rapid result may be available within 2 days, but complete karyotype results from cultured cells take on an average of 8–14 days. When performed at a high-volume, experienced center, the procedure-related pregnancy loss rate for amniocentesis and CVS is estimated to range from approximately one in 300 to one in 1,000 (0.1–0.3%).[11] The observed pregnancy loss rate after CVS is higher than after amniocentesis because CVS is performed at an earlier gestational age when the background risk for spontaneous loss is higher. Some studies suggest CMA as a first-line diagnostic test whenever fetal chromosomal analysis is indicated.[12] It provides more genetic information (e.g., microdeletions) than a conventional karyotype but is not more effective for diagnosis of Down syndrome and trisomy 18. It is more costly than a conventional karyotype.

Fluorescent in situ hybridization (FISH) targets chromosomes 13, 18, 21, X, and Y. FISH can be used for rapid diagnostic testing for common aneuploidies because it can be performed on interphase cells. Analysis of the full conventional karyotype/CMA is also performed to enable detection of other aneuploidies, as well as detection of major structural chromosomal abnormalities (e.g., translocations, inversions, and marker chromosomes) or microdeletions/duplications even if FISH is normal.

A quantitative fluorescence polymerase chain reaction (QF-PCR)-based approach is a recent rapid technique that can be used for rapid diagnostic testing detection of trisomies 13, 18, 21, X, and Y.[13-15] An added advantage of this technique is that it can be automated to allow high throughput of samples. As with FISH, analysis of the full karyotype/CMA needs to be performed if QF-PCR is normal and further information about fetal chromosomes is desired.

CONCLUSION

The widespread implementation of prenatal screening programs combined with prenatal diagnostic techniques and termination of affected pregnancy has substantially reduced the number of Down syndrome births.[16] In a systematic review of 24 United States studies (1995–2011) that reported data for pregnancies with confirmatory prenatal diagnosis of Down syndrome and subsequent pregnancy termination, the weighted mean termination rate was 67% (range 61–93%).[17]

It is important that the patient understands the exact purpose of screening tests and the difference between screening and diagnostic tests before they opt for that. The most important message is that a positive screen needs to be followed by a diagnostic test before any irreversible decisions are made. Likewise, patients need to understand that a negative screening test is not a foolproof guarantee. To achieve this end, patients along with their family members should be counseled on sensitivity, specificity, and positive predictive values of the available options of screening tests.[18] Identification of fetal anomalies and genetic conditions during the prenatal period allows parents and practitioners to prepare and opt for the right option. This could mean emotionally and socially preparing for a child with special needs, planning for delivery in a hospital best able to meet the neonate's needs, or terminating a pregnancy.[19]

REFERENCES

1. Ghosh K, Colah R, Manglani M, Choudhry VP, Verma I, Madan N, et al. Guidelines for screening, diagnosis and management of hemoglobinopathies. Indian J Hum Genet. 2014;20:101-19.
2. Phadke S, Agarwal M. Neural tube defects: a need for population-based prevention program. Indian J Hum Genet. 2012;18:145-7.
3. Central Technical Co-ordinating Unit, ICMR Central Technical Co-ordinating Unit, ICMR. Multicentric study of efficacy of periconceptional folic acid containing vitamin supplementation in prevention of open neural tube defects from India. Indian J Med Res. 2000;112:206-11.
4. Aggarwal S, Bogula VR, Mandal K, Kumar R, Phadke SR. Aetiologic spectrum of mental retardation & developmental delay in India. Indian J Med Res. 2012;136:436-44.
5. Uptodate.com/contents/down-syndrome-overview-of-prenatal-screening?csi=7818dda7-a7a5-433c-ac70-f3c75e9 f34e0&source=contentShare#H2959825032.
6. Gil MM, Quezada MS, Revello R, Akolekar R, Nicolaides KH. Analysis of cell-free DNA in maternal blood in screening for fetal aneuploidies: updated meta-analysis. Ultrasound Obstet Gynecol. 2015;45(3):249-66.
7. Hackshaw AK, Wald NJ. Repeat testing in antenatal screening for Down syndrome using dimeric inhibin-A in combination with other maternal serum markers. Prenat Diagn. 2001;21(1):58-61.
8. Bianchi DW, Parker RL, Wentworth J, Madankumar R, Saffer C, Das AF, et al. DNA sequencing versus standard prenatal aneuploidy screening. N Engl J Med. 2014;370(9):799-808.
9. Norton ME, Jacobsson B, Swamy GK, Laurent LC, Ranzini AC, Brar H, et al. Cell-free DNA analysis for noninvasive examination of trisomy. N Engl J Med. 2015;372(17):1589-97.
10. Palomaki GE, Kloza EM, O'Brien BM, Eklund EE, Lambert-Messerlian GM. The clinical utility of DNA-based screening for fetal aneuploidy by primary obstetrical care providers in the general pregnancy population. Genet Med. 2017; 19(7):778-86.
11. American College of Obstetricians and Gynecologists' Committee on Practice Bulletins—Obstetrics, Committee on Genetics, Society for Maternal–Fetal Medicine. Practice Bulletin No. 162: Prenatal Diagnostic Testing for Genetic Disorders. Obstet Gynecol 2016; 127:e108.
12. Fiorentino F, Napoletano S, Caiazzo F, Sessa M, Bono S, Spizzichino L, et al. Chromosomal microarray analysis as a first-line test in pregnancies with a priori low risk for the detection of submicroscopic chromosomal abnormalities. Eur J Hum Genet. 2013;21(7):725-30.
13. Mann K, Petek E, Pertl B. Prenatal detection of chromosome aneuploidy by quantitative fluorescence PCR. Methods Mol Biol. 2019;1885:139-60.
14. Masoudzadeh N, Teimourian S. Comparison of quantitative fluorescent polymerase chain reaction and karyotype analysis for prenatal screening of chromosomal

aneuploidies in 270 amniotic fluid samples. J Perinat Med. 2019;47(6):631-6.
15. Mann K, Hills A, Donaghue C, Thomas H, Ogilvie CM. Quantitative fluorescence PCR analysis of >40,000 prenatal samples for the rapid diagnosis of trisomies 13, 18 and 21 and monosomy X. Prenat Diagn. 2012;32(12):1197-204.
16. Palomaki GE, Chiu RWK, Pertile MD, Sistermans EA, Yaron Y, Vermeesch JR, et al. International Society for Prenatal Diagnosis Position Statement: cell free (cf)DNA screening for Down syndrome in multiple pregnancies. Prenat Diagn. 2021;41(10):1222-32.
17. Natoli JL, Ackerman DL, Mcdermott S, Edward JG. Prenatal diagnosis of down syndrome: A systematic review of termination rates (1995-2011). Prenat Diagn. 2012;32(2): 142-53.
18. https://www.ncbi.nlm.nih.gov/books/NBK557702/
19. Dukhovny S, Norton ME. What are the goals of prenatal genetic testing? Semin Perinatol. 2018;42(5):270-4.

Genetics and Counseling in Hemoglobinopathies

Megha Kamalapurkar, Vaishnavi PK

INTRODUCTION

The disorders of hemoglobin are broadly classified in to two groups—*hemoglobinopathies* and *thalassemias*.

Hemoglobinopathies are characterized by production of structurally defective hemoglobin due to abnormal production in globin moiety of the molecule (structurally abnormal hemoglobin).

Thalassemias are characterized by a reduced rate of production of normal hemoglobin due to absent or decreased synthesis of one or more types of globin polypeptide chains.

INCIDENCE

Hemoglobinopathies are common inherited disorders of hemoglobin affecting about 7% of the world population. Thalassemia is the most common single-gene disorder in India. The incidence of thalassemia is very high, with over 30 million people carrying the defective gene. Carrier frequency varies from 3 to 17% in different populations.[1]

The two important considerations for hemoglobinopathies during pregnancy are as following:
1. First screening for inheritance of abnormal globin genes needs to be considered in the potential offspring.
2. Second, physiological stress of pregnancy can worsen the hemoglobinopathy/thalassemia major syndrome which needs team approach, monitoring, and proper intervention to ensure the maternal and fetal safety.

The structure of hemoglobin is reviewed here before the hemoglobinopathies are described.

NORMAL HEMOGLOBIN

Normal human adult red blood cells contain three types of hemoglobin. They are hemoglobin A (HbA), hemoglobin A_2 (HbA$_2$), and fetal hemoglobin (HbF) **(Table 1)**.

Hemoglobin A comprises about 97% of hemoglobin of adult red cells. It consists of two alpha and two beta chains with structural formula $\alpha_2\beta_2$. Small amount of HbA are detected in fetus as early as the 8 week of fetal life. The switch of fetal Hb to adult HbA occurs by approximately 3–6 months after birth.

Hemoglobin A_2 is minor hemoglobin in adult red cell. It has a structural formula of alpha two delta two ($\alpha_2\delta_2$). HbA$_2$ is present in very small amounts at birth and reaches its adult level of 1.5–3.2% during the first year of life. Elevation of HbA$_2$ is a feature of some types of thalassemia and occasionally occurs in megaloblastic anemia and unstable hemoglobin disease. HbA$_2$ may be reduced in iron deficiency anemia.

Hemoglobin F ($\alpha_2\gamma_2$) is seen in fetal life. At term HbF accounts for 70–90% of total hemoglobin. It then rapidly falls up to 25% at 1 month and 5% at 6 months.

Hemoglobin Bart's is found in small amounts in cord blood if sensitive techniques are used.

CLASSIFICATION

Hemoglobinopathies are classified as minor and major and an intermediate form in between. Minor forms are asymptomatic and do not have any clinical phenotype whereas major forms present as a clinically significant disease.

Sickle Cell Anemia

In sickle cell anemia the higher amounts of HbF continue till 4 months of age. With gradual decline of HbF, sickle hemoglobin (HbS) levels increase with resultant formation of insoluble polymers that cause the typical sickle cell shape of RBCs that is characteristic of sickle cell anemia. This can cause significant morbidity and mortality in first 5 years of life.

TABLE 1: Types of hemoglobins with their structures, levels at birth, and levels in adults.				
Hemoglobin	Structure	Levels at birth	Levels in adults	Comments
A	$\alpha_2\beta_2$	20–25%	97%	Reaches adult level by 1 year of age
A_2	$\alpha_2\delta_2$	0.5%	2.5%	Elevated in beta thalassemia trait
F	$\alpha_2\gamma_2$	75–85%	<1%	Reaches adult level by 1 year of age
HbH	β_4	15–20% in HbH disease	NA	HbH produces Heinz bodies in the RBCs and hemolysis
Hb Barts	γ_4	100% in hydrops fetalis 15–20% in HbH disease	NA	Increased in carriers of alpha thalassemia traits at birth

Early identification has led to successful programs of vaccination and antibiotic prophylaxis and has helped reduce morbidity.

Due to sickle shape of red cells chronic intravascular and extravascular hemolysis occurs. These red cells have reduced life span and when red cells hemolyze, free hemoglobin is released resulting in endothelial activation and vasoconstriction that increases the risk of thrombosis (arterial or venous), vaso-occlusive crisis, or chronic hemolysis.

Sickle cell anemia refers to homozygous state where the child has inherited HbS from both the parents (Hb SS). HbS can also be coinherited with abnormal Hb resulting in a compound heterozygous state. These can also manifest as sickle cell anemia and couples should receive counseling about a possible sickle cell anemia phenotype with the following combination with HbS: HbSC, HbSB thalassemia, HbSD-Punjab, HbSO Arab, HbSE, and HbS Lepore.

Sickle cell trait, i.e., carrying a single *HbS* gene does not cause significant disease and is only noteworthy to trigger partner testing to determine the existence of HbS or any of the above abnormal hemoglobinopathies.

Thalassemia

Thalassemias are recessively inherited genetic disorders which affect the hemoglobin quantity produced in the body. This is due to changes in genetic code that regulated the production of alpha and beta chains of globin molecule.
- Alpha thalassemia major which is clinically significant to fetus and mother.
- Beta thalassemia that is clinically relevant after birth.
- Thalassemia intermedia which has a variable significance.

Alpha thalassemia: Normal HbA has two globin chains, however the production of these alpha globin chains is controlled by four alpha globin genes—two from each parent. The defect or mutation in one or more of the alpha globin genes results in either reduced or absent production of alpha globin chains.

The carrier status of alpha thalassemia can only be confirmed by deoxyribonucleic acid (DNA) analysis.

The normal graphic illustration of the alpha globin chains and full complement of alpha globin genes (four) that each individual with normal HbA inherits, this is usually written as $\alpha\alpha/\alpha\alpha$.

Alpha Thalassemia Major

In alpha thalassemia major (α^0) also known as Barts hydrops fetalis, there are no functioning alpha globin chains (–/–). As a result no globin chains are produced which results in life-threatening severe anemia in fetus and is fatal without intervention.

Alpha zero thalassemia carrier: This occurs when an individual has inherited no alpha globin chain genes from one of the parents (–/$\alpha\alpha$). This individual is healthy as there is only reduction in alpha globin chain production and may have mild anemia. Mean corpuscular hemoglobin (MCH) is usually <25 pg. It can be confused with iron deficiency anemia. If a couple are both carriers of alpha zero thalassemia carriers, then their carrier status must be identified by DNA analysis as there is 25% risk to all the children of inheriting the Barts hydrops fetalis, also known as alpha thalassemia major.

Alpha Plus Thalassemia

Individuals with alpha plus (α^+) thalassemia have inherited either one or two faulty alpha globin genes (-α/$\alpha\alpha$) or (-α/-α). Although this can affect alpha globin chain production, there is usually minimal change to the hemoglobin levels.

Alpha plus thalassemia is not clinically significant but can be confused with anemia in the antenatal period.

Hemoglobin H disease: A person with HbH disease (–/-α) has only one alpha globin gene but usually retains the ability to produce sufficient hemoglobin for life.

Beta Thalassemia Major

Beta thalassemia major is also called Cooley's anemia or Mediterranean anemia. This is most common in people of Pakistan, Italy, Greek, India, Bangladesh, China, etc.

Depending upon the beta thalassemia gene mutation inherited; there are three types of beta thalassemia as following:
1. Thalassemia minor (heterozygous β-thalassemia) with mild, microcytic, and hypochromic anemia.
2. Thalassemia intermedia (mild homozygous or mixed heterozygous β-thalassemia) of moderate severity and with a varying need for transfusions; typical complications are skeletal deformities and tumorous masses as a result of massive hyperplastic erythropoiesis.
3. Thalassemia major (severe homozygous or mixed heterozygous β-thalassemia) with long-term, transfusion-dependent anemia; untreated children die before the age of 10 years.

■ SCREENING OF HEMOGLOBINOPATHIES

The main objective of prenatal screening is to identify the couples at risk of having a child with sickle cell disease or thalassemia major syndrome and it should be a universal screening for all pregnant women. This is to provide the couple the option of continuing or terminating an affected pregnancy. The screening results need to be obtained in a timely manner to allow adequate counseling and fetal testing if required.

Screening programs first need to identify at risk couples. Ideally, screening should be universal.

■ HOW TO DO SCREENING?

The screening for hemoglobinopathies can be offered in stepwise manner **(Flowchart 1)**.

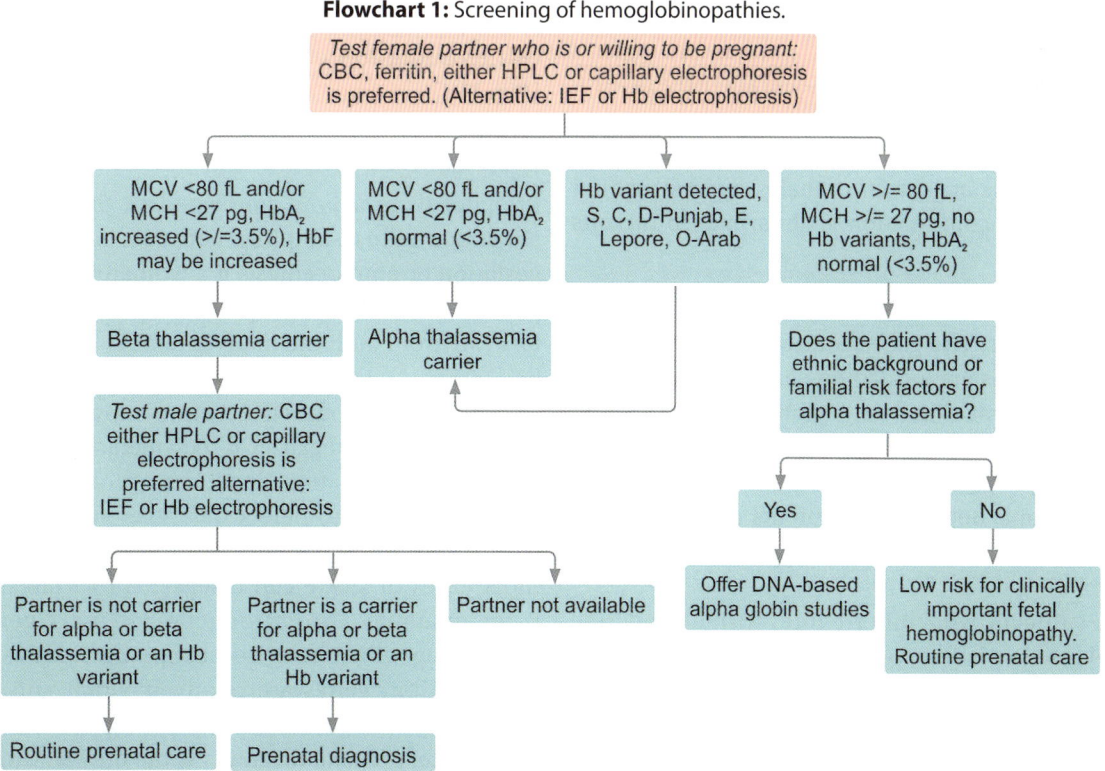

Flowchart 1: Screening of hemoglobinopathies.

(CBC: complete blood count; HPLC: high performance liquid chromatography; IEF: isoelectric focusing; MCH: mean corpuscular hemoglobin; MCV: mean corpuscular volume)

Step One: Universal Screening for All Pregnant Women

Thalassemia screening ideally should be offered to all pregnant women in public and private health sector.

Blood tests done for screening include complete blood count and peripheral smear that includes the measurement of a mean corpuscular volume (MCV) and/or MCH. Patients with decreased hemoglobin levels, low MCV and MCH in the absence of iron deficiency may have a form of thalassemia.

Hemoglobin electrophoresis [high performance liquid chromatography (HPLC)] is then performed to measure levels of hemoglobin including HbA, HbA_2, HbF, HbS as well as the other abnormal hemoglobin variants. Sickle cell trait can only be excluded if HbEP is normal.

Step Two: Screening

If a woman is found to have thalassemia trait (minor) her husband is advised to undergo the screening in same way as that of a pregnant lady. The carrier status of husband will decide further management options.

Step Three: Counseling for Hemoglobinopathies

Couples should be thoroughly counseled about the disease morbidity and mortality, inheritance pattern, options available so as help them take the informed decision. If both the partners are carrier of thalassemia/structural variant, molecular confirmation of abnormal Hb variants is advised.

Genetic regulation: Hemoglobinopathies are autosomal recessive disorders. The genes controlling production of alpha globin chains are located on chromosome number 16 and those controlling beta globin production on chromosome number 11. Everyone carries two copies (alleles) of HBB gene from each parent. HBB alleles are co-dominant. Beta-globin proteins are made from both alleles, and they combine randomly to make hemoglobin.

Thus subjects who inherit one normal and one abnormal gene are heterozygotes and those who have two identical abnormal genes are homozygotes. Double heterozygotes are subjects who have inherited two different abnormal genes. The homozygous state is usually referred as the disease and the heterozygous state as the trait.

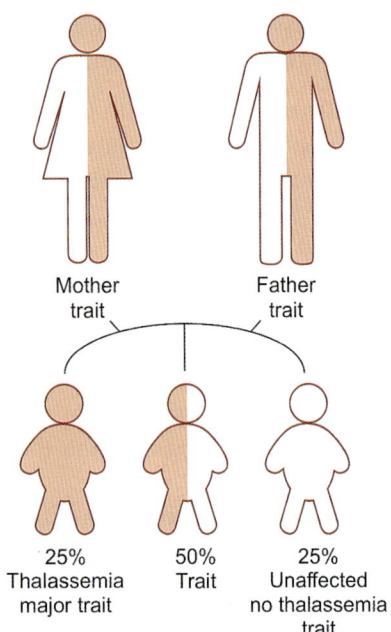

Fig. 1: Chances that the child will be a thalassemia patient, thalassemia carrier, or normal.

If both the partners are carriers for every pregnancy, there is a 25% chance that the child will be a thalassemia patient, a 50% chance that the child will be a thalassemia carrier, and a 25% chance that the child will be normal **(Fig. 1)**.

Step Four: Prenatal Diagnosis

Prenatal diagnosis is confirmed in first trimester by chorionic villus sampling between 10 and 12 weeks gestation or amniocentesis if a woman is at 15 weeks or greater in gestation. The procedure-related risk for fetal loss rate from both the interventions is of approximately 0.5–1.0%.

Confirmation by DNA sequencing of the α- and β-globin genes and gap-PCR (polymerase chain reaction) and multiplex ligation-dependent probe amplification (MLPA) analysis to detect deletions and duplications, is effective for screening and definitive diagnosis of most cases of sickle cell disease, Hb variants, α- and β-thalassemia. The introduction of next generation sequencing will probably not change much to this concept as the globin genes are relatively small and covered completely by direct Sanger sequencing.

To date, prenatal diagnosis is the only way to prevent the birth of an affected child. Therefore, in highly prevalent regions, an ideal and effective strategy to decrease the birth rate of thalassemia patients is to identify high-risk couples, who are both carriers, before pregnancy by screening (or carrier testing) and then perform a prenatal diagnosis during pregnancy.

Preimplantation genetic diagnosis may be available for families in which disease-causing mutations have been identified.[2]

■ CONCLUSION

Hemoglobinopathies are one of the preventable common genetic diseases. The prevention steps include, universal screening for pregnant women for carrier status. Prenatal genetic counseling: extended, husband and family screening if a woman is found to be a carrier. Prenatal diagnosis is done by preimplantation genetic tests, invasive tests as chorionic villous sampling or amniocentesis.

■ REFERENCES

1. Modell B, Bulzhenov V. Distribution and control of some genetic disorders. World Health Stat. 1988;41(3-4): 209-18.
2. Saxena R, Pati HP, Mahapatra M, Firkin F, Chesterman C, Penington D, et al. De Gruchy's Clinical Haematology in Medical Practice. 6th edition. India: Wiley India Pvt Ltd; 2012.

8

Common Congenital Fetal Anomalies and Genetic Associations

Vandana Bansal, Meera Jayaprakash

■ INTRODUCTION

The detection of congenital anomalies on ultrasound may prompt the clinician or the fetal medicine specialist to look for certain genetic associations which may be responsible for the condition. The relationship between the anomaly and the genetic test applied, however may not always be one-to-one. As of today, the field of genetics is an expanding one, with lists of pathogenic genes being updated on a daily basis, worldwide. A gene or chromosomal defect that seems to be responsible for a particular condition may, in the best-case scenario, correlate with the clinical findings. Conversely, it is possible that the congenital anomaly may not be associated with the most common genetic or chromosomal defect associated with the anomaly. Hence, genetic counseling is highly nuanced and riddled with riders, and it requires a judicious application of a test or a battery of tests to arrive at a diagnosis of a particular condition.

FIRST TRIMESTER NUCHAL TRANSLUCENCY AND ANOMALY SCAN

Nuchal translucency (NT) is an objective evaluation on ultrasound of subcutaneous fluid behind the fetal head, neck, and torso in the first trimester of pregnancy between 11^{+0} and 13^{+6} weeks of gestation, equivalent to a crown rump length of 45–84 mm **(Fig. 1)**. Increased NT thickness (above 95th centile) has been found to be associated with fetal chromosomal defects and in approximately 80% of fetuses with trisomy 21. NT is also increased in other conditions such as congenital heart defects, exomphalos, congenital diaphragmatic hernia, etc., and in many genetic and nongenetic syndromes.[1]

Double marker test includes maternal serum free beta human chorionic gonadotropin (β-hCG) and pregnancy-associated plasma protein A (PAPP-A), both produced by

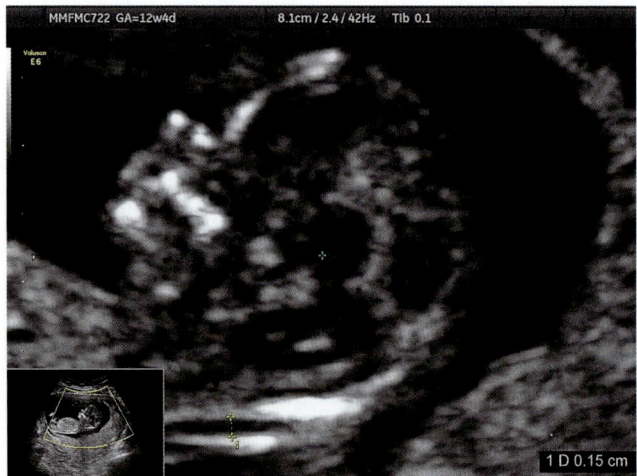

Fig. 1: Nuchal translucency.

placenta. Maternal serum concentration of free β-hCG (human chorionic gonadotropin) is higher (2 MOM) and PAPP-A is lower (0.5 MOM) in fetuses with trisomy 21. In trisomy 13 and 18 both free β-hCG and PAPP-A are decreased. In sex chromosomal anomalies only PAPP-A is low with normal free β-hCG.[2] Combined screen test is offered at $11-13^{+6}$ weeks of gestation which consists of maternal age, dual marker screen combined with NT. This gives a risk assessment for serious chromosomal anomalies, such as trisomy 21, 13, and 18. The detection rate of combined screen test for trisomy 21 is >90% for a 5% false-positive rate.

Addition of other first trimester markers (nasal bone/ductus venosus waveform/tricuspid regurgitation) increases detection rate for trisomy 21 to >95% for a false-positive rate of 2.5 and 95% with false-positive rate of 0.1% for trisomy 13 and 18. Nasal bone may not be visualized in 2% of chromosomally normal fetuses **(Figs. 2A and B)**. Abnormality of ductus venosus waveform is observed in 80% of trisomy 21 fetuses and 5% of euploid fetus.

Common Congenital Fetal Anomalies and Genetic Associations

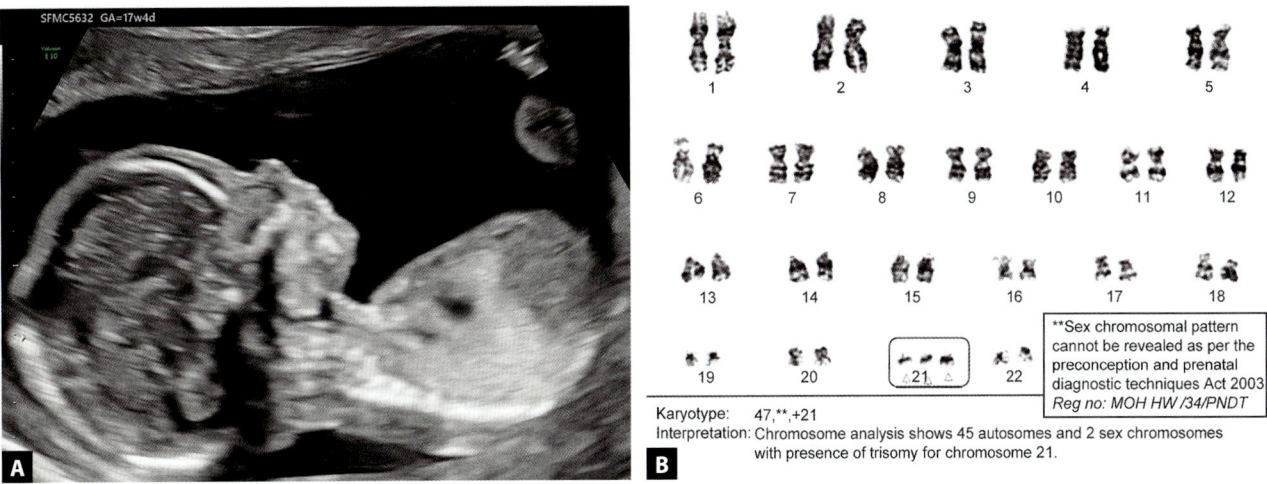

Figs. 2A and B: (A) Absent nasal bone; (B) Fetus with absent nasal bone with trisomy 21.

Tricuspid regurgitation is seen in 55% of trisomy 21 fetuses but also in 1% of normal fetuses. Abnormality of ductus venosus and tricuspid regurgitation may also be seen in fetuses with cardiac defects.[3]

Although the first trimester NT scan is done as a part of the screening protocol for Down syndrome, the scope can be extended to include the screening of certain anomalies. With the advances in imaging techniques and availability of better resolution ultrasound machines, it is becoming possible to detect major structural defects as early as in first trimester. Fetal malformations that can be reliably diagnosed at this gestation include anencephaly, holoprosencephaly, omphalocele, and limb defects.

An increased NT is a sensitive marker for the detection of Down syndrome, but it can also be a transient finding or it may be associated with other genetic syndromes and cardiac defects. In fetuses with increased NT, a detailed evaluation of the heart and major arteries in the first and second trimester along with the evaluation of blood flow across the tricuspid valve and in the ductus venosus can detect >90% of major congenital cardiac defects.[4] Increased NT is also associated with chromosomal abnormalities other than trisomy 21, like trisomy 18 and 13, Turner syndrome (45XO), Klinefelter syndrome (47XXY), other chromosomal trisomies and chromosomal translocations[5] which can be detected on a karyotype. In addition, some submicroscopic karyotypic abnormalities may also be associated with an increased NT, such as 22q11.2 deletion (DiGeorge/Velocardiofacial syndrome) among others.[6] Some single gene defects may also present with an increased NT. These include disorders such as lethal skeletal dysplasias, inborn errors of metabolism, fetal akinesia-deformation sequence and rasopathies like Noonan syndrome.[7] Thus, the cause of an increased NT can range from a karyotypic or submicroscopic karyotypic abnormality to a single gene defect. The preferred test, therefore, would depend either on the presence of other ultrasound abnormalities or on a significant positive history such as consanguinity or a family history of intellectual disability, infant or childhood morbidity or mortality or other genetic disorders. It would be prudent to suggest a chromosomal microarray at the outset along with deoxyribonucleic acid (DNA) storage for further testing, if the microarray is apparently normal.

Cystic hygroma, whether septate or not, is almost synonymous with an increased NT and is evaluated in a similar fashion.

SECOND TRIMESTER GENETIC SONOGRAM

A detailed ultrasonography (USG) for fetal anatomic survey is commonly used as an aneuploidy screening method in the second trimester which is usually best performed between 18 and 22 weeks gestation. Approximately one-third of fetuses affected with trisomy 21, have a major or minor structural variation identifiable on USG. Major abnormalities associated with Down syndrome are congenital heart defects, ventriculomegaly, and duodenal atresia.[8] Ultrasound abnormalities that have been associated with fetal aneuploidy other than Down syndrome are holoprosencephaly, facial cleft, cystic hygroma, diaphragmatic hernia, ventriculomegaly, posterior fossa cyst, major heart defects, duodenal atresia, omphalocele, early fetal growth restriction, and talipes.

Chromosomal defects associated with certain second trimester sonographic features (also known as soft markers), including biometric parameters (e.g., short length of femur and humerus, pyelectasis, increased nuchal fold thickness, ventriculomegaly, hypoplastic or absent nasal bone, early fetal growth restriction, and morphologic signs (e.g., choroid plexus cysts, echogenic bowel, echogenic and intracardiac focus). These "soft markers" are physical characteristics which are not themselves abnormalities or defects but occur more commonly in fetuses affected with aneuploidy.[9] By themselves or in isolation, they are usually not associated with fetal or neonatal morbidity or mortality.

The detection of any of the above markers during a routine sonogram warrants careful anatomical survey aimed at identifying additional markers because the finding of multiple markers indicates high risk for chromosomal anomaly. The soft markers that significantly increase the likelihood of trisomy 21 are thickened nuchal fold (measured in the transcerebellar plane) **(Fig. 3)**, mild ventriculomegaly, absent or hypoplastic nasal bone, echogenic bowel, and aberrant right subclavian artery. However, relying only on USG to identify Down syndrome is not recommended.

Genetic sonogram alone has a detection rate of 69% with a 5% false-positive rate and it enhances the sensitivity of all other screening methods. The pregnancy-specific risk of trisomy 21 is calculated by multiplying the *apriori* risk (maternal age and gestation dependent) by the likelihood ratio of each sonographic marker for the same pregnancy. The likelihood ratio is calculated by dividing the percentage of chromosomally abnormal fetuses by the percentage of chromosomally normal fetuses with the same measurement.[10]

The positive likelihood ratio for every marker present in fetus and the negative likelihood ratios of all the absent markers can be used to modify the apriori risk or serum screening risk which forms the basis for ultrasound screening for aneuploidy.[1,11] After the calculation of a pregnancy-specific risk, depending on the type of screening and their respective cut-off values, adequate post-test counseling is given to the patient regarding the requirement of an invasive test. For invasive testing, the sample is collected by amniocentesis, chorion villus sampling or by cordocentesis. It is on this sample that various tests are performed, depending on the indication of the test **(Table 1)**.

SECOND TRIMESTER STRUCTURAL ANOMALIES AND ASSOCIATION WITH GENETIC ABNORMALITIES

Universal ultrasound screening for fetal structural abnormalities is generally recommended at 18–22 weeks of gestational age. Screening for fetal cardiac malformations is part of routine ultrasound examination including the four-chamber view, outflow tracts, and three-vessel view. Few structural anomalies such as urinary tract abnormalities, microcephaly and skeletal dysplasia are progressive and late in onset and may not be detectable during the routine 18–20 weeks malformation scan.

Detecting major fetal structural anomalies in the second trimester (18–22 weeks) scan helps to identify abnormalities associated with severe morbidity or that are incompatible with life, so that couple can make an informed choice about termination of pregnancy within constraints of law. A scan at this gestational age also detects abnormalities which require early neonatal intervention or which may benefit from in-utero fetal therapeutic interventions.

There is a significant overlap between cardiac defects, structural anomalies, and genetic abnormalities. Hence there is a need for prenatal diagnostic testing whenever a structural anomaly is diagnosed antenatally. Chromosomal microarray analysis (CMA) is recommended for prenatal diagnosis in cases with one or more fetal structural abnormalities.

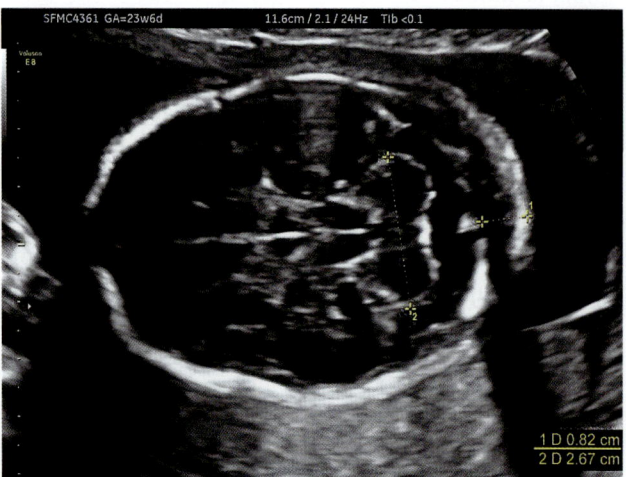

Fig. 3: Increased nuchal fold thickness.

TABLE 1: Tests that can be performed on a fetal sample for genetic diagnosis.

Test	Method	Turnaround time	Advantage	Limitation
Fluorescent in situ hybridization (FISH)	Fluorescent probe for certain chromosomes/suspected deletions used	24–48 hours	Rapid, does not require cell culture or metaphase cells, can detect mosaicism	Labor-intensive, does not test all chromosomes, cannot detect structural rearrangements
Quantitative fluorescent polymerase chain reaction (qf-PCR)	PCR using markers for certain chromosomes, read on an electrophoretogram	24–48 hours	Rapid, automated (less labor-intensive)	Does not test all chromosomes, cannot detect structural rearrangements
Karyotype	Cell culture, followed by analysis of chromosomes on metaphase cells by G-banding	10–14 days	Shows all chromosomes, including structural rearrangements and large deletions, can detect mosaicisms	Culture dependent, long turnaround time, labor-intensive
Chromosomal microarray	Detects gain or loss of genetic material by comparing with standard template, depending on depth of reading, different arrays can be tested	7–10 days	Submicroscopic changes in chromosomes can be detected depending on depth, algorithm-based	Cannot detect structural rearrangements, variants of uncertain significance
Sanger sequencing	Tests single gene with a known sequence	7–10 days	Cost-effective, especially if the pathogenic variant is known and the gene is sequenced	Tests only for specific genes or a gene panel
Multiplex ligation-dependent probe amplification (MLPA)	Tests variations in copy number of multiple genes, used for detection of deletions and duplications	3–7 days	• Can detect variants in multiple genes responsible for similar phenotype, e.g., Duchenne muscular dystrophy, spinal muscular atrophy • More cost-effective than Sanger sequencing	May not be able to detect loss of heterozygosity, may show problems in mosaicism
Clinical exome sequencing	Sequences the protein coding regions of disease-causing genes	10–28 days	Can detect variants in multiple genes, correlation with phenotype gives relevant results	Variants of uncertain significance, should be interpreted with caution, may detect pathogenic variants with late expressivity
Whole exome sequencing	Sequences the protein coding regions of >20,000 genes (~1–2% of genome)	10–28 days	Can detect variants in multiple genes, correlation with phenotype gives relevant results	Variants of uncertain significance, should be interpreted with caution, may detect pathogenic variants with late expressivity
Trio exome sequencing	Sequences the exome of the parents and the proband	10–28 days	Can detect variants in multiple genes, correlation with phenotype gives relevant results, more cost- and time-effective than exome of only proband	Variants of uncertain significance, should be interpreted with caution, may detect pathogenic variants with late expressivity
Whole genome sequencing	Sequences the whole genome, including the coding and noncoding regions	10–28 days	Can detect variants in multiple genes, more effective than exome sequencing, correlation with phenotype gives relevant results	Variants of uncertain significance, should be interpreted with caution, may detect pathogenic variants with late expressivity

CENTRAL NERVOUS SYSTEM

Holoprosencephaly is a severe brain abnormality caused by incomplete cleavage of the embryonic forebrain. Alobar holoprosencephaly is a first-trimester diagnosis which is picked up due to an inability to visualize the butterfly-shaped choroid plexuses. It is usually associated with severe ocular abnormalities such as a single eye (cyclopia) or closely set eyes (hypotelorism), nasal abnormalities such as absent nose (arrhinia) with a single proboscis (ethmocephaly) or a single nostril (cebocephaly), and midline palatal and facial clefts (**Figs. 4A and B**).

Alobar holoprosencephaly is usually associated with trisomy 13 (Patau syndrome). Submicroscopic karyotypic abnormalities, and single gene defects also have been implicated through various studies.[11,12] However, due to the lethal nature of alobar holoprosencephaly and the possibility of a relatively early diagnosis using ultrasound, a karyotype and DNA saved is the preferred test in order to determine the risk of recurrence of aneuploidy in subsequent pregnancies. Lobar holoprosencephaly on the other hand is diagnosed usually in the middle or late second trimester. Like alobar holoprosencephaly, lobar holoprosencephaly is also seen in chromosomal disorders, submicroscopic defects, and single gene defects.[13] Poor survival rate and the possibility of severe neurodevelopmental disorders should be explained to the couple along with option of termination of pregnancy.

Ventriculomegaly, defined as dilation of the fetal cerebral ventricles of >10 mm at any gestational age. When isolated it is a strong soft marker for aneuploidy with a likelihood ratio of 3.8. It may be a normal variant or marker for aneuploidy, genetic syndromes, primary brain or spinal abnormalities, congenital infection, cerebrovascular accidents, and intracranial hemorrhage.

Ventriculomegaly is a sign of an underlying disorder, and a careful evaluation is needed to arrive at a diagnosis. Ventriculomegaly may be seen in association with agenesis of corpus callosum, posterior fossa cystic lesions such as Dandy–Walker malformation, and with malformation of cortical development like lissencephaly. A careful history, fetal neurosonogram/fetal magnetic resonance imaging (MRI) and a detailed ultrasound for extracerebral abnormalities can help to arrive at a diagnosis. Amniocentesis is advisable for microarray and infection testing by TORCH PCR (toxoplasmosis, rubella, cytomegalovirus, and herpes simplex virus polymerase chain reaction) and DNA should be saved for detecting single gene disorders, if infectious etiology can be ruled out. The overall prognosis strongly depends on the extent of ventricular enlargement presence of other abnormal findings and progression of disease. Hence, it needs to be followed up for progression or appearance of associations. Asymmetric pattern is a potential risk factor for anomalies of neuropsychological development.

Posterior fossa cystic lesions may be transient like Blake's pouch cyst which usually disappears by the late second trimester; relatively benign like mega cisterna magna or they may be part of Dandy–Walker malformation and inferior vermian hypoplasia, which are associated with severe neuromotor disability.

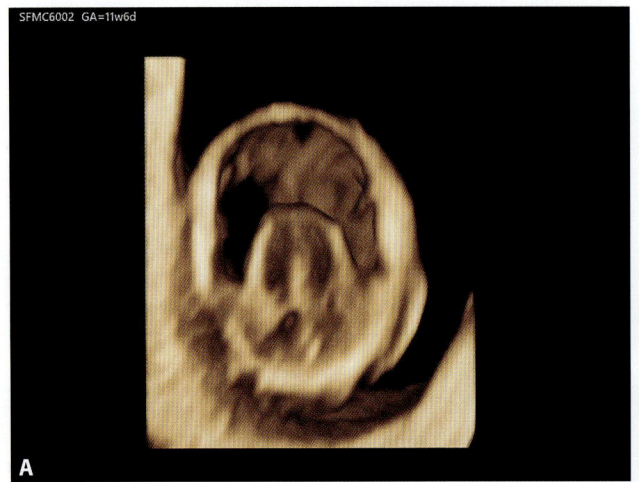
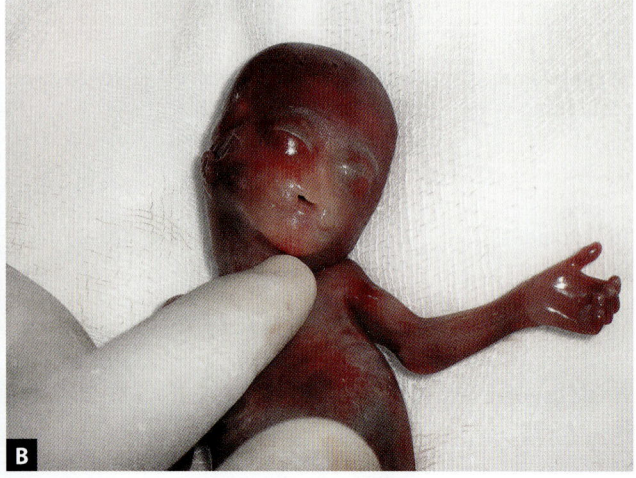

Figs. 4A and B: (A) Ultrasonography in the first trimester showing holoprosencephaly; (B) Abortus of holoprosencephaly with trisomy 13 with median cleft lip.

Dandy–Walker malformation is usually occurred due to chromosomal causes[14,15] or submicroscopic abnormalities[16] (**Figs. 5A and B**).

Increased NT with an open fourth ventricle with hypoplastic vermis with a molar tooth sign is suggestive of Joubert syndrome. These disorders together constitute an autosomal recessive group of genetic disorder called ciliopathies. Joubert syndrome presents as ataxia, developmental delay, abnormal eye movements, retinal coloboma, hyperechoic kidneys, and polydactyly. The other syndromes in this group include COACH (coloboma, oligophrenia, ataxia, cerebellar hypoplasia), CORS (cerebello-oculo-renal), and OFD VI (orofaciodigital). Joubert syndrome and related disorders are caused by multiple gene mutations. Genetic counseling and molecular diagnosis may be offered.[17]

Cerebellar hypoplasia is a small but normal looking cerebellum which may be a part of autosomal recessive neurodegenerative disorder named pontocerebellar hypoplasia. Molecular testing for the specific gene mutation is necessary in present and subsequent pregnancies for early prenatal diagnosis.

Occipital encephalocoele or cephaloceles in general are not associated with aneuploidy. However, they may be associated with other malformations and syndromes such as Apert, Walker Warburg, craniotelencephalic dysplasia, facio-auriculo-vertebral, and oculo-encephalo-hepato-renal syndromes. Commonest among all is a triad of polycystic kidneys, polydactyly, and encephalocele that is pathognomonic for Meckel–Gruber syndrome, an autosomal recessive disorder. Cephaloceles may also be associated with destructive lesions such as amniotic rupture sequence or limb-body wall complex, in which case a genetic test may not yield any results. A chromosomal microarray or a next-generation sequencing (NGS)-based test, depending on other ultrasound findings may be required to determine the cause of cephaloceles.[18]

Agenesis of corpus callosum (ACC) is essentially diagnosed in the second trimester, since the corpus callosum just begins to develop at 12 weeks and can be just seen by 14–15 weeks of gestation.[19] Certain screening tests have been described to screen for agenesis of corpus callosum in the first trimester,[20] but they are not routinely used. Though agenesis of corpus callosum by itself is not a lethal anomaly, when associated with other conditions such as ventriculomegaly, posterior fossa abnormalities, or lissencephaly, they may be the cause of intellectual disability, motor impairment, or seizure disorders.[21]

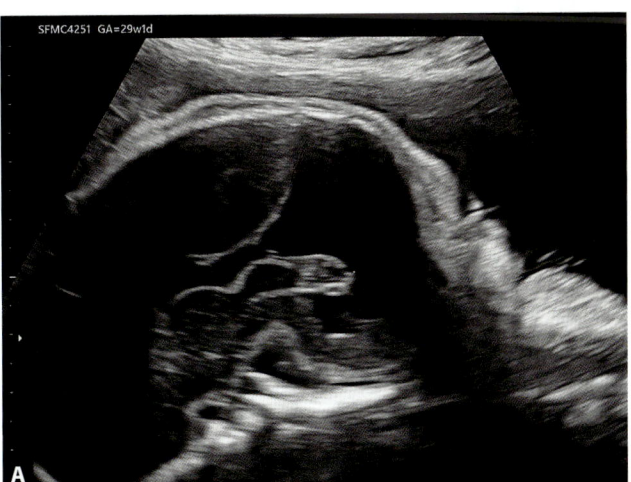

Likely pathogenic variant causative of the reported phenotype was detected						
Gene (Transcript)#	Location	Variant	Zygosity	Disease (OMIM)	Inheritance	Classification
TUBB (+) (ENST00000327892.8)	Exon 4	c.860C>T (p.Pro287Leu)	Heterozygous	Complex cortical dysplasia with other brain malformations-6	Autosomal dominant	Likely pathogenic

Figs. 5A and B: (A) Ultrasonography showing Dandy–Walker malformation; (B) Same fetus with Dandy–Walker malformation with a single gene disorder.

There is a wide genetic heterogeneity and agenesis of corpus callosum may be a part of a syndrome. Agenesis of corpus callosum with dysmorphic facies and polydactyly is suggestive of Acrocallosal syndrome (AR)[22] or orofacial digital syndrome which is X-linked dominant.[23] Aicardi syndrome is seen in females (X-linked recessive) with heterotropia, polymicrogyria, microphthalmia, hemivertebra along with ACC. It is lethal in male fetuses.[24] Diagnosis is by testing for the specific gene mutations or whole exome study.

Microcephaly (head circumference <-3SD) is a late diagnosis with high morbidity and high recurrence. It has a varied etiology and may be part of chromosomal aberrations, Mendelian syndrome, perinatal infections, inborn errors of metabolism (phenylketonuria) or prenatal exposure to drugs (aminopterin), alcohol abuse, malnutrition, or hypoxia.[25] Fetal chromosomal microarray, infection screening and molecular testing in the amniotic fluid should be considered to determine recurrence risk.

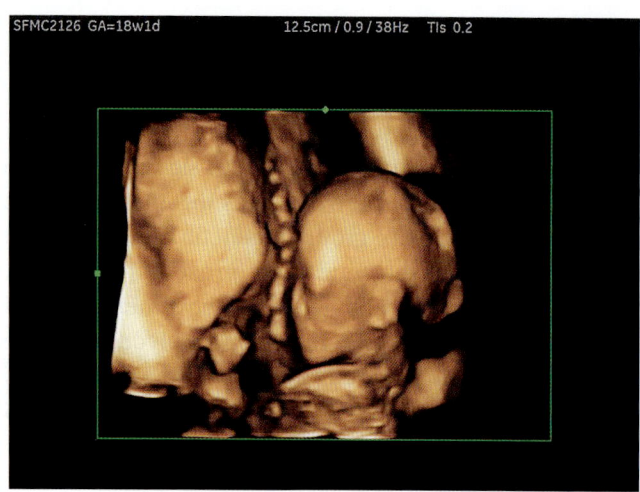

Fig. 6: Ultrasonography image of Binder facies.

■ FETAL FACE

An absent nasal bone in the first trimester (defined as nasal bone not seen, or its echogenicity being less than the overlying skin), or a hypoplastic nasal bone in the second trimester is a strong soft marker for aneuploidies. Maternal ethnicity is a factor, with absent nasal bones being higher in the Afro-Caribbean women as compared to Caucasians.[26] Aneuploidy can be diagnosed by karyotype. However, certain pathogenic submicroscopic abnormalities have also been reported in fetuses with absent nasal bone with additional abnormalities that can be detected by chromosomal microarray.[27]

Binder syndrome or maxillofacial dysplasia is a commonly observed ultrasound finding characterized by a flat nasal bridge **(Fig. 6)**. It is a mild form of skeletal dysplasia and may be multifactorial with etiologies ranging from maternal intake of coumarin-based anticoagulants, maternal lupus, or genetic syndromes.[28] The most commonly described genetic syndrome showing Binder facies is chondrodysplasia punctata.[29] It is usually caused by single gene defects which may be autosomal recessive or X linked. Inborn errors of metabolism and chromosomal disorders such as Turner syndrome may also show features of chondrodysplasia punctata.[30,31]

Cleft lip with or without cleft palate is a common anomaly picked up in the second trimester, though it may be picked up in the first trimester too.[32] The etiology for cleft lip and palate has been considered multifactorial, folate deficiency and maternal alcohol and smoking implicated as some causative factors.[33] Clefts may be unilateral, bilateral, or median. Midline cleft lip and palate may be seen in disorders of ventral induction like holoprosencephaly, especially the more severe versions **(Fig. 4B)**. Median clefts are associated with trisomy 13. Cleft lip and palate may be syndromic or isolated. Syndromes showing cleft lip and palate include ectrodactyly-ectodermal dysplasia-cleft (EEC) syndrome, Van der Woude syndrome, Wolf–Hirschhorn syndrome, and many others.[34,35] Nonsyndromic cleft lip and palate have many candidate genes which are considered pathogenic.[36] Identification of cleft lip with or without cleft palate should prompt a detailed evaluation of the fetus to rule out other abnormalities and fetal testing for chromosomal microarray.

■ FETAL ABDOMEN

Anterior abdominal wall defects include gastroschisis, omphalocele, and limb-body wall complex. Omphalocele results from failure of reversal of physiological herniation of bowel loops into the umbilical cord between 6 and 10 weeks of gestation.[37] It may contain bowel loops or a part of the liver. There is a high likelihood of aneuploidies in fetuses with small omphaloceles not containing the liver. Conversely, the omphaloceles containing part of the liver may have an apparently normal karyotype but may be associated with other fetal structural abnormalities[38] **(Fig. 7)**. Fetuses with an apparently normal karyotype may have submicroscopic abnormalities or single gene

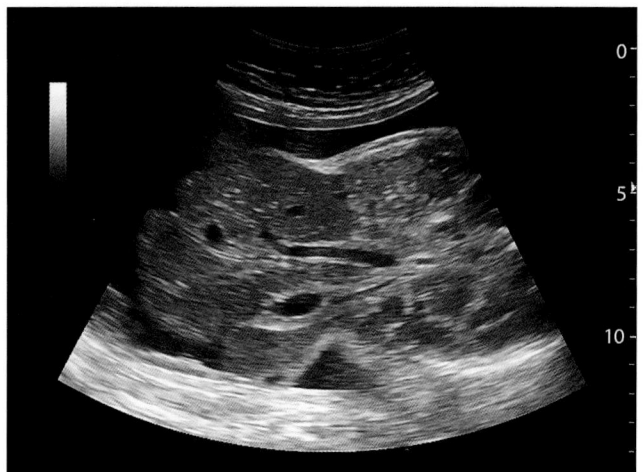

Fig. 7: Ultrasonography of large omphalocele with liver as content with normal karyotype.

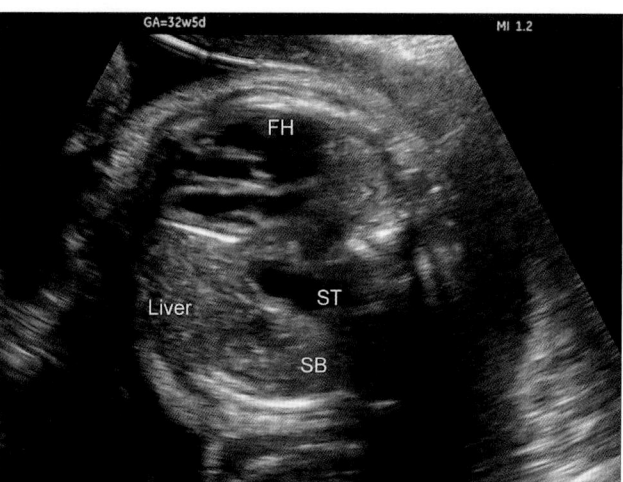

Fig. 8: Ultrasonography of a congenital diaphragmatic hernia with liver, small bowel, and stomach in the thorax.

disorders that may be diagnosed using microarray or NGS-based testing.[39]

While omphalocele is associated with a high risk of antenatal mortality due to its association with other congenital anomalies and chromosomal aneuploidies, an isolated omphalocele carries a good postsurgical prognosis in the neonatal period. On the other hand gastroschisis is not associated with other major anomalies or chromosomal aneuploidies but these neonates may have a complex postnatal period depending upon the extent of organ involvement. Limb-body wall complex and Pentalogy of Cantrell are universally lethal and not associated with genetic abnormalities and are mostly terminated. Antenatal detection of these anterior abdominal wall defects enables detailed prenatal planning, amniocentesis for chromosomal aneuploidy in omphalocele, antenatal monitoring for intestinal obstruction and appropriate intrauterine transfer, delivery in a tertiary referral center with prompt access to pediatric surgery, and early surgical intervention.

Diaphragmatic hernia is a herniation of abdominal contents into the thorax through an orifice in the diaphragm. Diaphragmatic hernias are usually diagnosed in the mid or the third trimester. However large hernias may be picked up in the first trimester. Diaphragmatic hernias may be isolated, or may be associated with multiple syndromes **(Fig. 8)**. The risk of recurrence of isolated diaphragmatic hernia is low.[40] Syndromic diaphragmatic hernia on the other hand, may be associated with chromosomal abnormalities, especially aneuploidies and translocations.[41] In addition, multiple microdeletion and duplication syndromes have also been associated with diaphragmatic hernia. Single gene disorders have also been described as causative for diaphragmatic hernia.[42]

Congenital diaphragmatic hernia is a malformation with important implications due to high mortality. Prognosis is poor with early gestation at diagnosis, associated liver herniation and a low lung to head circumference ratio (LHR <1). LHR is the ratio of opposite normal lung area to the head circumference at that gestation.[43] The mainstay of management includes meticulous initial evaluation of LHR and extent of liver herniation, chromosomal analysis, antenatal monitoring of the fetus for signs of worsening, cardiac dysfunction and development of hydrops under expert fetomaternal unit care, delivery near term at a tertiary care center with NICU set-up, standard protocols for management of neonate at birth including initial intubation, stabilization and treatment of pulmonary hypertension and then surgical management.[44]

CONGENITAL LUNG MALFORMATIONS

Fetal thoracic masses include congenital pulmonary adenomatoid malformation (CPAM) and broncho-pulmonary sequestration (BPS), are multifactorial and do not need prenatal genetic testing. Both of these fetal lung masses when associated with hydrops are nearly 100% fatal.[45] Congenital pulmonary airway malformation volume ratio (CVR) helps determine the risk of development of hydrops and is an important parameter which is to be considered when counseling such patients. CVR is the volume of the CPAM mass normalized for gestational age. A CVR >1.6 or a CPAM with a dominant large cyst increases risk of developing hydrops.[46] The natural history of this lung lesion may be progression/regression or remains stable antenatally and hence require monitoring prenatally. In the postnatal period, early thoracoscopic surgery (between 4 and 6 months) is indicated if neonate is symptomatic, with few pre- and postoperative complications, limited chest deformation during growth and limited impact on pulmonary growth and low parental anxiety.[47]

■ FETAL GASTROINTESTINAL ANOMALIES

Intestinal atresia is a common cause of neonatal obstruction, secondary to mesenteric vascular accidents during intrauterine life. The most common type is esophageal atresia, followed by atresia in the jejunoileal region and in the duodenum.[48] Higher the obstruction earlier is the time of presentation in antenatal period by visualization of polyhydramnios and dilated bowel loops proximal to the obstruction. Prenatal diagnosis of bowel obstruction and referral to tertiary center with early neonatal surgical correction reduces morbidity due to aspiration pneumonia or further abdominal distention with respiratory embarrassment if undiagnosed.[49]

The "double-bubble" sign on ultrasound is a marker for duodenal atresia, usually seen in fetuses with trisomy 21 **(Fig. 9)**. However, it may also be seen in heterotaxy syndromes, intestinal malrotations, and

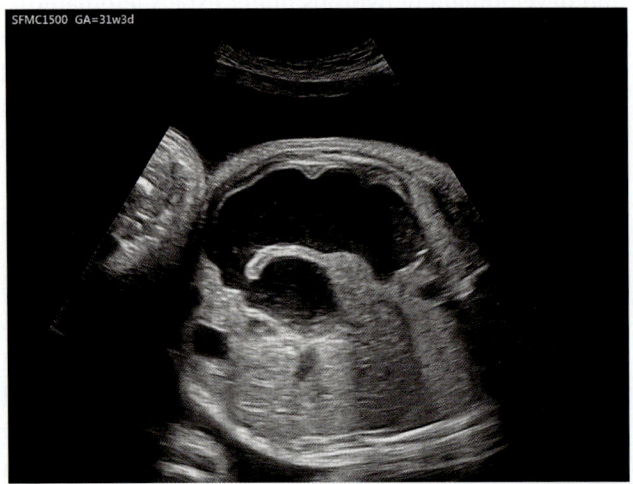

Fig. 9: Ultrasonography of double bubble sign with communication suggestive of duodenal atresia.

certain microdeletion syndromes.[50] Lower small bowel obstructions are usually not associated with genetic abnormality.

Anorectal atresia (ARA) is a major congenital malformation and it is frequently associated with other anomalies. An association between vertebral, anal, cardiovascular, tracheoesophageal, renal, and limb malformations has been recognized and termed the VACTERL syndrome.[51] Anorectal anomalies are also found frequently in association with sacral agenesis and lower limb hypoplasia as part of the caudal regression syndrome.[52]

■ SKELETAL SYSTEM

Skeletal dysplasias are a wide and varied group of bony abnormalities that can affect any part of the skeleton. It may range from mild conditions like Binder syndrome to severe abnormalities like osteogenesis imperfecta and lethal ones like thanatophoric dysplasia. The more lethal skeletal disorders can usually be recognized on ultrasound in the first or the early second trimesters. The milder and nonlethal abnormalities usually present in the late mid-trimester or third trimester. Skeletal dysplasias are usually single gene disorders. One of the most common skeletal dysplasias is achondroplasia, which can be recognized by short femur and humerus length, defined as the respective lengths less than the 5th centile for gestational age.[53] A short humerus and femur may also be seen in aneuploidies like trisomy 21.[54] Achondroplasia, thanatophoric dysplasia, and certain other skeletal dysplasias are due to mutations in the *FGFR3* gene. However, skeletal dysplasias show a wide genotypic and phenotypic heterogeneity. A narrow thorax, polyhydramnios, fetal hydrops, etc., are usually associated with lethality.[55] Fetal club hand or radial ray deformity can be a marker for chromosomal aneuploidies, single gene defects and Fanconi anemia.[56] NGS-based testing may be required for fetuses with an apparently normal karyotype.

■ FETAL GENITOURINARY ANOMALIES

Urinary tract dilatation disorders include pelviureteric junction obstruction, vesicoureteric reflux or obstruction, posterior urethral valves, urethral atresia. All of these present with varying grades of hydronephrosis with/without hydroureter and/or oligohydramnios, depending upon the severity of obstruction, and level of obstruction. All urinary tract dilatations require 3–4 weekly antenatal monitoring for worsening, oligohydramnios, cortical thickness, and echogenicity so as to decide time of delivery balancing the risk of prematurity versus worsening renal function. These disorders are usually multifactorial.[57] Pyelectasis is also considered a soft marker for aneuploidy, albeit with a low likelihood ratio.

Autosomal dominant polycystic kidney may be diagnosed in the third trimester as enlarged kidneys, with or without the presence of cysts, but with the urinary bladder visible. Oligohydramnios is rarely a feature. In contrast, autosomal recessive polycystic kidney disease may be diagnosed in the first or early second trimester with enlarged kidneys with poor corticomedullary differentiation and severe oligo- or anhydramnios.[58] These follow the Mendelian inheritance pattern and need to be confirmed in the index case.

Multicystic kidney disease refers to the presence of noncommunicating large renal cysts. This may be a progressive abnormality and may be seen in the late second or even the third trimester. It may be multifactorial or associated with single gene abnormalities such as ciliopathies.[59]

Renal agenesis, whether unilateral or bilateral, may be associated with numerous single gene syndromes.[60] It is necessary to have a detailed evaluation of the fetus to rule out other anomalies. In the case of bilateral renal agenesis, this may not be possible due to severe oligo- or anhydramnios. Bilateral renal agenesis has a poor prognosis owing to pulmonary hypoplasia as a result of anhydramnios.

Megacystis, defined as a fetal urinary bladder size >7 mm in the first trimester, is associated with chromosomal aneuploidies specially trisomy 18. Aneuploidies may be present regardless of fetal bladder size; hence karyotype can be offered in all cases of fetal megacystis.[61] Megacystis may also be observed in bladder outlet obstruction, overgrowth syndromes such as Beckwith-Wiedemann and Sotos syndrome, or may be associated with Megacystis microcolon intestinal hypoperistalsis (MMIH) syndrome.[62]

■ FETAL HEART

Congenital heart disease is the most common congenital anomaly, affecting about 1% of the population.[63] An evaluation of the fetal heart along with markers such as tricuspid valve and ductus venosus flow can help detect certain major cardiac anomalies in the first trimester itself.

Certain anomalies such as endocardial cushion defect, perimembranous ventricular septal defects, and tetralogy of Fallot **(Fig. 10)** are seen antenatally in Down syndrome, whereas coarctation of aorta and hypoplastic left heart syndrome may be seen in fetuses with Turner syndrome.[64] Conotruncal anomalies such as common arterial trunk, interrupted aortic arch, tetralogy of Fallot, double outlet right ventricle, transposition of great arteries, etc., may be seen in cases with 22q11.2 deletions (DiGeorge syndrome).[65] Heterotaxy syndromes and situs abnormalities usually are caused by single gene defects such as ciliopathies. There is a considerable degree of overlap of the cardiac abnormality with the extracardiac disorder involved. For instance, though heterotaxy syndromes have been shown to be mostly single-gene disorders, they have also been associated with aneuploidies, chromosomal rearrangements[66] and with microarray abnormalities.[67] Hence, a detailed evaluation of the fetus to determine the nature of cardiac anomaly along with a search for extracardiac abnormalities may help to direct investigations.

Cardiac rhabdomyoma, which is usually seen in the late second or the third trimester is almost pathognomonic of tuberous sclerosis,[68] although sporadic rhabdomyomas have also been reported. A detailed family history of seizures, renal disorders, and cardiac arrhythmia along with renal ultrasound of the parents to detect renal angiomyolipomas should be undertaken. Tuberous sclerosis complex is caused by autosomal dominant pathogenic mutations in the *TSC1* or *TSC2* genes with

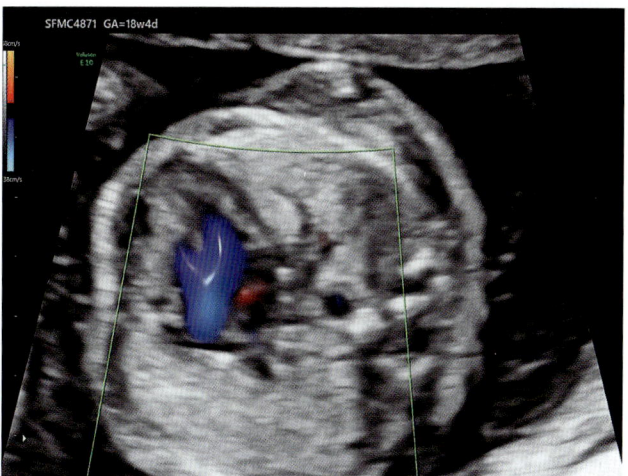

Fig. 10: Ultrasonography of an 18-week fetus with Fallot's tetralogy.

a recurrence of 50% if one of the parents is carrying the affected gene. It is a multisystem disorder, and though not uniformly fatal, is a cause of morbidity.

CONCLUSION

Obstetricians, fetal medicine specialists, geneticists, neonatologists, pediatric surgeons, and other specialists frequently need to counsel parents about the implications of a prenatally diagnosed ultrasound finding. This provides the affected families with valuable insights into the need for delivery in an appropriate setting, by the safest mode of delivery, at the gestational age appropriate to minimize effects of the anomaly, and surgical management of the anomaly. Additionally need for genetic testing and its implications to the overall survival and morbidity of the fetus as well as recurrence risk in next pregnancy must be understood.

Certain anomalies that may be detected by ultrasound do not warrant genetic testing. These include acrania-exencephaly-anencephaly sequence, fetal open neural tube defects, gastroschisis, limb reduction defects, isolated single umbilical artery, cystic pulmonary and airway malformations, bronchopulmonary sequestration, posterior urethral valves, and limb-body wall complex abnormalities.

Genetic disorders are varied and a single genotype may show multiple phenotypes and vice versa. The knowledge of the genetic etiologies of these anomalies as well as the tests required to arrive at a genetic diagnosis helps to complete the puzzle. It can help to prognosticate, both in the case of the incumbent pregnancy as well as in subsequent pregnancies. In addition, it can help to guide treatment.

The expertise of a geneticist is invaluable in such cases, whereby they not only help to narrow down the causative factors, but also suggest the appropriate tests to arrive at a diagnosis. Probably in the future, with the help of gene-editing technologies, the knowledge of the genetic etiology of diseases may help to completely cure certain genetic conditions which are considered incurable at present. A high index of suspicion while performing ultrasound, a multidisciplinary approach, and a detailed knowledge of the genetic syndromes and causative genes help to address the root cause of abnormalities and help the couple to take an informed decision, for the present pregnancy as well as in the future.

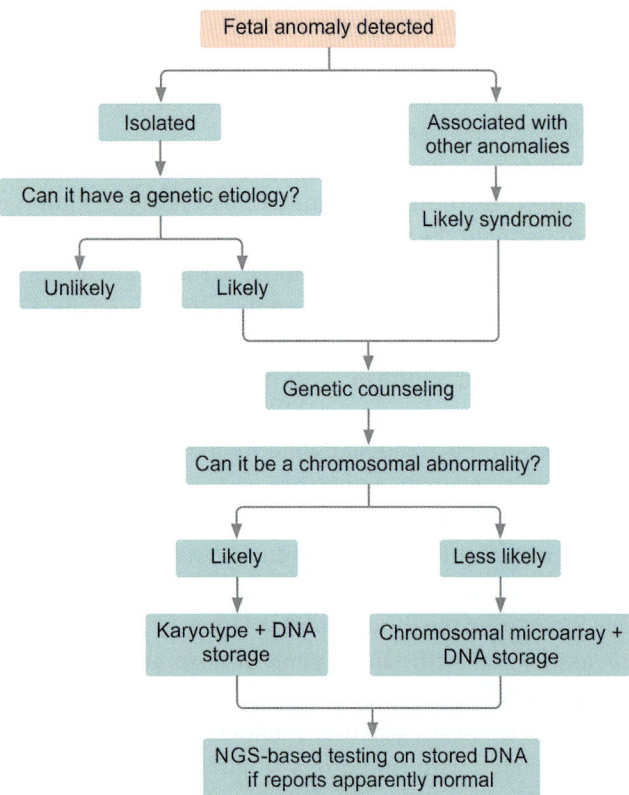

Flowchart 1: Prenatal diagnosis and genetic evaluation for structural defects.

DNA: deoxyribonucleic acid; NGS-based: next-generation sequencing based

Since different congenital anomalies have different etiologies, this algorithm may not be the final word in the diagnostic process, but it can help to put things in perspective **(Flowchart 1)**.

REFERENCES

1. Bhide A, Arulkumaran S, Damania KR, Daftary SN. Chapter 1: Prenatal diagnosis of chromosomal abnormalities. In: Arias F, Bhide AG, Arulkumaran S, Damania K, Daftary SN (Eds). Arias' Practical guide to high risk pregnancy and delivery—A south Asian perspective. 4th edition. India: Elsevier; 2015. pp. 1-12
2. Snijders RJM, Nicolaides KH. Chapter 1: First trimester diagnosis of chromosomal defects. In: Snijders R, Nicolaides K (Eds). The 11-13^{+6} Weeks Scan. 1st edition. London: Fetal Medicine Foundation; 2004. pp. 7-58.
3. Nicolaides KH. Nuchal translucency and other first-trimester sonographic markers of chromosomal abnormalities. Am J Obstet Gynecol. 2004;191:45-67.
4. Minnella GP, Crupano FM, Syngelaki A, Zidere V, Akolekar R, Nicolaides KH. Diagnosis of major heart defects by

routine first-trimester ultrasound examination: association with increased nuchal translucency, tricuspid regurgitation and abnormal flow in ductus venosus. Ultrasound Obstet Gynecol. 2020;55:637-44.
5. Müller MA, Pajkrt E, Bleker OP, Bonsel GJ, Bilardo CM. Disappearance of enlarged nuchal translucency before 14 weeks' gestation: relationship with chromosomal abnormalities and pregnancy outcome. Ultrasound Obstet Gynecol. 2004;24:169-74.
6. Leung TY, Vogel I, Lau TK, Chong W, Hyett JA, Petersen OB, et al. Identification of submicroscopic chromosomal aberrations in fetuses with increased nuchal translucency and apparently normal karyotype. Ultrasound Obstet Gynecol. 2011;38:314-9.
7. Souka AP, Snijders RJ, Novakov A, Soares W, Nicolaides KH. Defects and syndromes in chromosomally normal fetuses with increased nuchal translucency thickness at 10-14 weeks of gestation. Ultrasound Obstet Gynecol. 1998;11(6):391-400.
8. Norton ME, Scoutt LM, Feldstein VA. Chapter 3: Ultrasound evaluation of fetal aneuploidy in the first and second trimesters. In: Callen's Ultrasonography in Obstetrics and Gynecology. 6th edition. Philadelphia: Elsevier; 2017. pp. 57-77.
9. Snijders RJM, Nicolaides KH. Sequential screening. In: Nicolaides KH (Ed). Ultrasound Markers for Fetal Chromosomal Defects. Carnforth, UK: Parthenon Publishing; 1996. pp. 109-13.
10. Nicolaides KH. Screening for fetal aneuploidies at 11 to 13 weeks. Prenat Diagn. 2011;31(1):7-15.
11. Croen LA, Shaw GM, Lammer EJ. Holoprosencephaly: epidemiologic and clinical characteristics of a California population. Am J Med Genet. 1996;64:465-72.
12. Belloni E, Muenke M, Roessler E, Traverso G, Siegel-Bartelt J, Frumkin A, et al. Identification of Sonic hedgehog as a candidate gene responsible for holoprosencephaly. Nat Genet. 1996;14(3):353-6.
13. Tekendo-Ngongang C, Muenke M, Kruszka P. Holoprosencephaly overview. In: Adam MP, Mirzaa GM, Pagon RA, Wallace SE, Bean LJH, Gripp KW, et al. (Eds). GeneReviews®. Seattle (WA): University of Washington, Seattle; 2000.
14. Imataka G, Yamanouchi H, Arisaka O. Dandy-Walker syndrome and chromosomal abnormalities. Congenit Anom. 2007;47(4):113-8.
15. Sun Y, Wang T, Zhang N, Zhang P, Li Y. Clinical features and genetic analysis of Dandy-Walker syndrome. BMC Pregnancy Childbirth. 2023;23(1):40.
16. Shaffer LG, Rosenfeld JA, Dabell MP, Coppinger J, Bandholz AM, Ellison JW, et al. Detection rates of clinically significant genomic alterations by microarray analysis for specific anomalies detected by ultrasound. Prenat Diagn. 2012;32(10):986-95.
17. Parisi M, Glass I. Joubert syndrome. In: Adam MP, Mirzaa GM, Pagon RA, Wallace SE, Bean LJH, Gripp KW, et al. (Eds). GeneReviews®. Seattle (WA): University of Washington, Seattle; 2003.
18. Sepulveda W, Wong AE, Andreeva E, Odegova N, Martinez-Ten P, Meagher S. Sonographic spectrum of first-trimester fetal cephalocele: review of 35 cases. Ultrasound Obstet Gynecol. 2015;46(1):29-33.
19. De León Reyes NS, Bragg-Gonzalo L, Nieto M. Development and plasticity of the corpus callosum. Development. 2020;147(18):189738.
20. Kalaycı H, Tarım E, Özdemir H, Çok T, Parlakgümüş A. Is the presence of corpus callosum predictable in the first trimester? J Obstet Gynaecol. 2018;38(3):310-5.
21. Palmer EE, Mowat D. Agenesis of the corpus callosum: a clinical approach to diagnosis. Am J Med Genet C Semin Med Genet. 2014;166C(2):184-97.
22. Putoux A, Thomas S, Coene KLM, Davis EE, Alanay Y, Ogur G, et al. KIF7 mutations cause fetal hydrolethalus and acrocallosal syndromes. Nat Genet. 2011;43(6):601-6.
23. Slavotinek AM, Chao R, Vacik T, Yahyavi M, Abouzeid H, Bardakjian T, et al. VAX1 mutation associated with microphthalmia, corpus callosum agenesis, and orofacial clefting: the first description of a VAX1 phenotype in humans. Hum Mutat. 2012;33(2):364-8.
24. Sutton VR, Van den Veyver IB. Aicardi syndrome. In: Adam MP, Mirzaa GM, Pagon RA, Wallace SE, Bean LJH, Gripp KW, et al. (Eds). GeneReviews®. Seattle (WA): University of Washington, Seattle; 2006.
25. Becerra-Solano LE, Mateos-Sánchez L, López-Muñoz E. Microcephaly, an etiopathogenic vision. Pediatr Neonatol. 2021;62(4):354-60.
26. Cicero S, Sonek JD, Mckenna DS, Croom CS, Johnson L, Nicolaides KH. Nasal bone hypoplasia in trisomy 21 at 15–22 weeks' gestation. Ultrasound Obstet. Gynecol. 2003;21(1):15-8.
27. Dukhovny S, Wilkins-Haug L, Shipp T, Benson CB, Kaimal AJ, Reiss R. Absent fetal nasal bone: what does it mean for the euploid fetus? J Ultrasound Med. 2013;32(12):2131-4.
28. Keppler-Noreuil KM, Wenzel TJ. Binder phenotype: associated findings and etiologic mechanisms. J Craniofac Surg. 2010;5:1339-45.
29. Sheffield LJ, Halliday JL, Jensen F. Maxillonasal dysplasia (Binder's syndrome) and chondrodysplasia punctata. J Med Genet. 1991;28:503-4.
30. Irving MD, Chitty LS, Mansour S, Hall CM. Chondrodysplasia punctata: a clinical diagnostic and radiological review. Clin Dysmorph. 2008;17(4):229-41.
31. Morrisom SC. Punctate epiphyses associated with Turner syndrome. Pediatr Radiol. 1999;29:478-80.
32. Lakshmy SR, Deepa S, Rose N, Mookan S, Agnees J. First-trimester sonographic evaluation of palatine clefts: a novel diagnostic approach. J Ultrasound Med. 2017;36(7):1397-414.

33. Murray J. Gene/environment causes of cleft lip and/or palate. Clin Genet. 2002;61:248-56.
34. Van der Woude A. Fistula labii inferioris congenita and its association with cleft lip and palate. Am J Hum Genet. 1954;6:244-56.
35. Morishita M, Shiba R, Chiyo H, Furuyama J, Fujita H, Atsumi Y. The oral manifestations of 4p-syndrome. J Oral Maxillofac Surg. 1983;41:601-5.
36. Aylward A, Cai Y, Lee A, Blue E, Rabinowitz D, Haddad J Jr, et al. Using whole exome sequencing to identify candidate genes with rare variants in nonsyndromic cleft lip and palate. Genet Epidemiol. 2016;40(5):432-41.
37. Sadler TW. Body cavities. In: TW Sadler (Ed). Langman's Medical Embryology. Lippincott, Williams and Wilkins: Baltimore, MD, USA; 2010. pp. 155-64.
38. Khalil A, Arnaoutoglou C, Pacilli M, Szabo A, David AL, Pandya P. Outcome of fetal exomphalos diagnosed at 11-14 weeks of gestation. Ultrasound Obstet Gynecol, 2012;39:401-6.
39. Shi X, Tang H, Lu J, Yang X, Ding H, Wu J. Prenatal genetic diagnosis of omphalocele by karyotyping, chromosomal microarray analysis and exome sequencing. Ann Med. 2021;53(1):1285-91.
40. Pober BR, Lin A, Russell M, Ackerman KG, Chakravorty S, Strauss B, et al. Infants with Bochdalek diaphragmatic hernia: sibling precurrence and monozygotic twin discordance in a hospital-based malformation surveillance program. Am J Med Genet A. 2005;138A(2):81-8.
41. Tibboel D, Gaag AV. Etiologic and genetic factors in congenital diaphragmatic hernia. Clin Perinatol. 1996;23(4):689-699.
42. Holder AM, Klaassens M, Tibboel D, de Klein A, Lee B, Scott DA. Genetic factors in congenital diaphragmatic hernia. Am J Hum Genet. 2007;80(5):825-45.
43. Jani J, Nicolaides KH, Keller RL, Benachi A, Peralta CF, Favre R, et al. Observed to expected lung area to head circumference ratio in the prediction of survival in fetuses with isolated diaphragmatic hernia. Ultrasound Obstet Gynecol. 2007;30(1):67-71.
44. Alfaraj MA, Shah PS, Bohn D, Pantazi S, O'Brien K, Chiu PP, et al. Congenital diaphragmatic hernia: lung-to-head ratio and lung volume for prediction of outcome. Am J Obstet Gynecol. 2011;205(1):43.e1-8.
45. Cass DL, Olutoye OO, Cassady CI, Moise KJ, Johnson A, Papanna R, et al. Prenatal diagnosis and outcome of fetal lung masses. J Pediatr Surg. 2011;46(2):292-8.
46. Crombleholme TM, Coleman B, Hedrick H, Liechty K, Howell L, Flake AW, et al. Cystic adenomatoid malformation volume ratio predicts outcome in prenatally diagnosed cystic adenomatoid malformation of the lung. J Pediatr Surg. 2002;37(3):331-8.
47. Adzick NS, Flake AW, Crombleholme TM. Management of congenital lung lesions. Sem Pediatr Surg. 2003;12:10-6.
48. Aguayo P, Ostile DJ. Duodenal and intestinal atresia and stenosis. In: Holcomb GW, Murphy JP, Ostlie DJ (Eds) Ashcraft's Pediatric Surgery. 6th edition, Philadelphia: Elsevier; 2014.
49. Hemming V, Rankin J. Small intestinal atresia in a defined population: occurrence, prenatal diagnosis and survival. Prenat Diagn. 2007;27(13):1205-11.
50. Bishop JC, McCormick B, Johnson CT, Miller J, Jelin E, Blakemore K, et al. The double bubble sign: duodenal atresia and associated genetic etiologies. Fetal Diagn Ther. 2020;47(2):98-103.
51. Rittler M, Paz JE, Castilla EE. VACTERL association, epidemiologic definition and delineation. Am J Med Genet. 1996;63:529-36.
52. Kylat RI, Bader M. Caudal Regression Syndrome. Children (Basel). 2020;7(11):211.
53. Papageorghiou AT, Fratelli N, Leslie K, Thilaganathan B. Outcome of fetuses with antenatally diagnosed short femur. Ultrasound Obstet Gynecol. 2008;31:507-11.
54. Brumfield CG, Hauth JC, Cloud GA, Davis RO, Henson BV, Cosper P. Sonographic measurements and ratios in fetuses with Down syndrome. Obstet Gynecol. 1989;73(4):644-6.
55. Krakow D, Lachman RS, Rimoin DL. Guidelines for the prenatal diagnosis of fetal skeletal dysplasias. Genet Med. 2009;11(2):127-33.
56. Brons JTJ, van der Harten HJ, van Geijn HP, Wladimiroff JW, Niermeijer MF, Lindhout D, et al. Prenatal ultrasonographic diagnosis of radial-ray reduction malformations. Prenat Diagn. 1990;10:279-88.
57. Nguyen HT, Benson CB, Bromley B, Campbell JB, Chow J, Coleman B, et al. Multidisciplinary consensus on the classification of prenatal and postnatal urinary tract dilation (UTD classification system). J Pediatr Urol. 2014;10(6):982-98.
58. Talati AN, Webster CM, Vora NL. Prenatal genetic considerations of congenital anomalies of the kidney and urinary tract (CAKUT). Prenat Diagn. 2019;39(9):679-92.
59. Kagan KO, Dufke A, Gembruch U. Renal cystic disease and associated ciliopathies. Curr Opin Obstet Gynecol. 2017;29(2):85-94.
60. Deshpande C, Hennekam RCM. Genetic syndromes and prenatally detected renal anomalies. Semin Fetal Neonatal Med. 2008;13(3):171-80.
61. Lesieur E, Barrois M, Bourdon M, Blanc J, Loeuillet L, Delteil C, et al. Megacystis in the first trimester of pregnancy: Prognostic factors and perinatal outcomes. PLoS One. 2021;16(9):e0255890.
62. Fontanella F, Maggio L, Verheij JBGM, Duin LK, Adama Van Scheltema PN, Cohen-Overbeek TE, et al. Fetal megacystis: a lot more than LUTO. Ultrasound Obstet Gynecol. 2019;53(6):779-87.
63. van der Linde D, Konings EE, Slager MA, Witsenburg M, Helbing WA, Takkenberg JJ, et al. Birth prevalence of congenital heart disease worldwide: a systematic review and meta-analysis. J Am Coll Cardiol. 2011;58:2241-7.
64. Pierpont ME, Brueckner M, Chung WK, Garg V, Lacro RV, McGuire AL, et al. Genetic Basis for Congenital Heart

Disease: Revisited: A Scientific Statement From the American Heart Association [published correction appears in Circulation. 2018 Nov 20;138(21):e713]. Circulation. 2018;138(21):e653-711.
65. Marino B, Digilio MC, Toscano A, Anaclerio S, Giannotti A, Feltri C, et al. Anatomic patterns of conotruncal defects associated with deletion 22q11. Genet Med. 2001;3:45-8.
66. Sutherland MJ, Ware SM. Disorders of left-right asymmetry: heterotaxy and situs inversus. Am J Med Genet C Semin Med Genet. 2009;151C(4):307-17.
67. Cowan JR, Tariq M, Shaw C, Rao M, Belmont JW, Lalani SR, et al. Copy number variation as a genetic basis for heterotaxy and heterotaxy-spectrum congenital heart defects. Philos Trans R Soc Lond B Biol Sci. 2016;371(1710): 20150406.
68. Kocabaş A, Ekici F, Cetin Iİ, Emir S, Demir HA, Arı ME, Değerliyurt A, Güven A. Cardiac rhabdomyomas associated with tuberous sclerosis complex in 11 children: presentation to outcome. Pediatr Hematol Oncol. 2013;30(2):71-9.

9 Genetics and Infertility

Shovandeb Kalapahar, Sujoy Dasgupta

■ INTRODUCTION

Among the different factors causing infertility, genetics is the most complex one. Many important aspects of fertility such as gonadal development, gametogenesis, synthesis of hormones etc. are basically controlled by multiple genes. So, it is imperative to have in depth knowledge in genetics to treat infertility.

■ GENETICS IN FEMALE INFERTILITY

Embryonic development depends upon the euploidy status of genome and on different cytoplasmic components. Various genes control multiple biological process involved in oogenesis, control of ovarian aging, signaling pathways of hormones, and development of reproductive organs in female and also its functionality. Alteration of these controlling genes causes female infertility by large abnormalities of chromosomes, deletion and duplications of genes and also variation of deoxyribonucleic acid (DNA) sequences.

Role of genetics in female infertility can be divided into different subgroups:

Female Sexual Development

It has been found that karyotypes are normal (46XX) in 92% of women with Müllerian anomalies and abnormal in 7.7% of these women. Mutation in *HOXA10* and *HOXA11* genes has been identified in patients with uterine malformations. Various congenital uterine malformations, such as including Mayer-Rokitansky-Kuster-Hauser syndrome[1] are reported to be associated with heterozygous variants of different genes—*LHX1*, *HNF1B*, *WNT4*, *WNT7A*, and *WNT9B*.

X Chromosome and Female Infertility

Accelerated loss of primordial oocytes during female fetal development is observed resulting in streak gonads at birth.[2,3] That ultimately leads to premature ovarian insufficiency (POI).[4] Chromosomal abnormalities (*monosomy X—Turner syndrome*), balanced and unbalanced X-autosome rearrangements of X autosome (mosaicism) and also deletion and duplications of genes (*BMP15*, *FMR1*, and *PGRMC1*) are responsible for this. An entire X chromosome with karyotype of 45XO is seen in about 50% of affected women. About 20% have varying degrees of mosaicism, mostly 45,XO/46XX karyotype[5] and also 25% have a partially deleted one X-chromosome. XY cell line is also seen in about 5% of affected women. Ultrasonographically detected ovaries are seen in 26% of affected girls with 45X karyotypes, whereas in mosaic Turner patients, two detectable larger volume ovaries are seen in 76% of patients. Spontaneous thelarche (50%) and menarche (38.5%) are observed in girls with mosaicism more frequently than those with 45X karyotypes. Individuals with 45X karyotypes are reported to conceive spontaneously and delivering healthy infants; though women with mosaicism are more likely to conceive spontaneously. Among Turner syndromes, who conceive spontaneously used to carry mosaic karyotypes in >90% of women.[6]

XY Gonadal Dysgenesis

Swyer syndrome usually presents as female appearing external genitalia and Müllerian structure with XY chromosomes, lack of spontaneous pubertal development, absent breast development, dysgenic and nonfunctional gonads leading to primary amenorrhea and infertility. Deletions or pathogenic sequence alterations affecting the SRY gene on the Y chromosome have been observed in approximately 10-15% of XY gonadal dysgenesis.[7-9]

Androgen Insensitivity Syndrome

Mutation in the intracellular androgen receptor genes with 46XY karyotype (located on the long arm of the

X chromosome) leads to female phenotype—well developed breast but short blind vagina with primary amenorrhea.

XX Gonadal Dysgenesis

Type of alteration (gain vs. loss of function) that affects specific protein domains determines phenotypic expression and severity of impaired gonadogenesis. Segregation defects can alter oogenesis leading to female infertility. POI can also be the result of defect in DNA damage repair gene that causes accelerated apoptosis. Meiotic nondisjunction and aneuploidy associated with aging leading to infertility.[10] It can also be due to gradual loss of cohesions or cohesion-related proteins such as *SGO2*. Nonsyndromic primary ovarian insufficiency may be due to accelerated loss of oocyte with unrepaired double strand DNA breaks. It is mainly due to deficiency of DNA repair genes such as *MCM8*, *MCM9*, *MSH5*, and *XRCC4*.[11-13]

Maternal-effect factors necessary for embryonic activation are regulated by different oocyte-specific transcription factors; such as NOBOX, LHX8, FIGLA, SOH LH1, and SOH LH2. They also control follicular development and play a role in cytoplasmic maturation.[14]

Hypogonadotropic hypogonadism is relatively uncommon presentation with deficiency of gonadotropin-releasing hormone (GnRH) hormone due to its impaired production or defects in secretion or function. In almost 50% of patients with hypogonadotropic hypogonadism, Kallmann syndrome is observed.

Normal maturation of oocytes depends upon follicle-stimulating hormone (FSH) and its receptor's gene. Further maturation of preantral stages is blocked due to pathogenic variants in FSHβ (FSH beta subunit) and FSHR (FSH receptor) genes. Changes in FSHR cause hypergonadotropic hypogonadism,[15] whereas defects in FSHβ lead to less production of FSH, leading to hypogonadotropic hypogonadism.[16] Defects in the formation of zona pellucida and subsequent infertility may be due to nucleotide variations in genes of human zona pellucida.

Reproductive Aging

Premature ovarian insufficiency cases with no detectable FSH/LH receptor mutations show a deficit in ovarian follicles. These vary from complete failure of germ-cell development, resulting in primary amenorrhea, to an accelerated decline in germ cell numbers, leading to the cessation of ovarian function before age 40. Multiple genetic factors have been reported in such cases, including FOXL2, STAG3, FOXO3a, and X-linked genes, such as *FMR1* and *BMP15* located at Xp11.2. Among them fragile X mental retardation gene (*FMR1*), located at Xq27.3 needs to be mentioned. It involves trinucleotide (CGG) repeat sequence mutation. Normally *FMR1* gene contains approximately 30 repeats. Repeats between 55 and 200 are responsible for the disorder. The prevalence of premutation is approximately 15% among women with familial POI and lower, but still significant (1–7%), in those having no family history of POI.[17] All women with POI should be offered screening for the *FMR1* premutation.

Diminished Ovarian Reserve

Different regulatory genes such as *BMP15* and *GDF9* are involved in granulosa cell proliferation, cumulus expansion steroidogenesis, and apoptosis. These genes are the members of the transforming growth factor β (TGF β) superfamily. Transition from the primary to secondary follicle stage is also controlled by GDF9.[18] Heterozygous variants of *BMP15* and *GDF9* genes are involved up to 10% of hypergonadotropic hypogonadism.[19]

Multigenic Factors

Polycystic Ovary Syndrome

Susceptibility loci on chromosomes 9q33.3 and 2p16.3,2p21 are identified by genome wide association studies. Additional studies identify 16 independent signals in 15 genomic regions associated with polycystic ovary syndrome (PCOS) including signals near important reproductive hormone genes *FSHR*, *LHCGR*, and *FSHB*.

Endometriosis: The most recent meta-analysis identified 14 genomic regions associated with disease risk. Endometriosis is an estrogen-dependent disease and estrogen receptor 1 (ESR1) is the predominant receptor for estrogen action in the endometrium. Estrogen and progesterone receptor polymorphisms are important causative factors.

In Repeated Implantation Failure

Different genetic association also found in repeated implantation failure (RIF). Fertilization failure may be the result of failure to complete MII exit and pronuclei formation. This is due to pathogenic variants in *WEE2* gene. Meiotic spindle assembly in oocyte is essentially regulated by *TUB88* gene encoding a beta-tubulin subunit. Failure to form spindle or disorganized spindle and also defects in extrusion of polar body—these are due to pathogenic variation in *TUBB8*. Germinal vesicle arrest with primary infertility is the result of loss of function of PATL2. These are some causes of postfertilization preimplantation embryonic failure.[19]

Outline of Treatment

Peripheral blood karyotype is the basic investigation in clinically suspected female. Different gene sequencing method such as next generation sequencing (NGS) or whole exome sequencing (WES) is important to identify clinically relevant genetic variants. *FMR1* gene mutation should be performed in POI cases. PGD (now called preimplantation for monogenic disorder PGT-M) is helpful in identifying euploid embryo in known genetically affected individuals. But according to ESTEEM (Effect of Simple, Targeted Diet in Pregnant Women With Metabolic Risk Factors on Pregnancy Outcomes) trial 2017, evaluation of oocyte euploidy in general population with age group between 36 and 41 years by array CGH does not improve clinical outcome.

In Müllerian anomalies with absence of uterus, surrogacy is the only option. Whereas, in POI patients, donor egg IVF is the option. In hypogonadotropic hypogonadism, ovarian stimulation with human menopausal gonadotropin (HMG) followed by intrauterine insemination (IUI) or in vitro fertilization (IVF) is the treatment option.

In vitro fertilization with donor oocyte is the option for fertility treatment in Turner syndrome. Acceptable successful pregnancy rates of about 24–47% have been observed in women undergoing IVF, who do not have Turner syndrome.[3] Miscarriages are commonly found in women with Turner syndrome due to presence of hypoplastic uterus with thin endometrium.[20] Single embryo transfer is recommended in smaller uterus of Turner syndrome to reduce complications. Recently autologous IVF has been reported in women with Turner syndrome, who have functional ovaries. Normal serum FSH and AMH levels, spontaneous puberty with mosaic karyotype are the predictors for successful autologous IVF. Whereas structurally anomalous X chromosome or monosomy, elevated FSH levels, low AMH levels, lack of spontaneous puberty are the negative predictors for successful autologous IVF.[21]

Fertility preservation is important in these patients, but timing for it is controversial. Oocyte or ovarian tissue cryopreservation in adolescents (before ovarian failure) and reproductive aged women have been reported in several case reports.[22] Although, safety of these procedures in prepubertal females has not been confirmed. Effect of these treatments on adult height or on other pubertal development is unknown. Ovarian wedge resection by laparoscopy with subsequent cryopreservation is an alternative option.

■ GENETICS OF MALE INFERTILITY

In male, the fertility potential requires proper functioning of the testes themselves, the hypothalamo-pituitary axis and the outflow tract. All of them are controlled by several genes.

Testicular Failure

The common genetic causes are structural and numerical abnormalities of sex chromosomes and deletion of genes located in Y chromosome.

Sex chromosome abnormalities: The most common congenital cause of hypogonadism in male is *Klinefelter's syndrome* (KS) with incidence 1:1,000 male birth.[23] KS is also the commonest sex chromosomal abnormality associated with azoospermia.[23,24] The usual karyotype is 47,XXY but sometimes mosaic (46,XY/47,XXY) or additional X chromosome (48,XXXY) have also been reported.[23] This syndrome is also seen in males having translocation of the testis-determining gene (SRY) leading to the karyotype of 46,XX. The underlying factor is the nondisjunction of the sex chromosomes during meiosis. The cause of nonobstructive azoospermia (NOA) is because of atrophy of seminiferous tubules, and damage of germ cells and Leydig cells.[23] It leads to hypergonadotropic hypogonadism.[23]

In men with KS, particularly those with mosaic form, low levels of spermatogenesis can be present inside the testicles.[23] Such sperms can be recovered by testicular sperm extraction (TESE) or preferably with microscopic TESE (micro-TESE) and can be utilized for intracytoplasmic sperm injection (ICSI).[23] With such techniques, spermatozoa can be retrieved from 50% men with KS, leading to pregnancy, and live birth rate of 50%.[25] However, the babies born out of these procedures are at risk of having 47,XXY abnormalities because of presence of sperms carrying abnormalities in sex chromosomes (24,XY sperms) and autosomes (disomy for chromosomes 13, 18, and 21).[23] Therefore, sperms obtained from KS men should be checked for aneuploidy by sperm fluorescent in situ hybridization (FISH) and if appropriate, preimplantation genetic testing (PGT) should be offered.[23]

Y chromosome cluster mutation: Y chromosome gene mutations are the commonest "molecular genetic cause" of severe male factor-infertility.[23] The region azoospermia factor (AZF), present in the long arm of Y chromosome (Yq), contains several genes controlling the spermatogenesis (24). Deletions involving this region remove one or more of the genes partially or completely and are known as Y-chromosome microdeletion (YMD).[23] YMD is not found in men with normozoospermia and is extremely rare in men with sperm concentration >5 million/mL.[23] The prevalence of such defect is 3–7% in men with severe oligospermia and 8–12% in men with azoospermia.[23] The most common variety is AZFc deletion followed by deletions of AZFb, AZFb + c, and AZFa + b + c.[23] AZFa complete microdeletion causes Sertoli cell-only syndrome whereas that of AZZFb causes spermatogenetic arrest.[23] On the other hand AZFc deletion can be associated with oligospermia or azoospermia.[23] Men with azoospermia and oligospermia (concentration <5 million/mL) should be offered genetic testing for YMD and if such deletions are detected, genetic counseling should be done, because of the risk of transmission from father to son.[23] Even the offsprings are at risk of developing Turner's syndrome (45,XO) and ambiguous genitalia.[23] Apart from YMD, a new type of Y chromosome deletion known as the "gr/gr deletion" has been described, which can predispose to oligospermia and testicular tumors.[23]

Other genetic problems: In infertile male, karyotype may sometimes reveal 46,XX pattern because of DNA translocation from part of Y chromosome to X chromosome. In contrast, 46,XY male can have disorders of sexual development (DSD) because of enzyme deficiency (17,20 desmolase, 17-α-hydroxysteroid dehydrogenase) and gonadal dysgenesis (due to various genetic mutations). Leydig cell hypoplasia because of inactivating LH receptor mutations can also cause spermatogenetic failure.

Hypothalamo-pituitary Dysfunction

Just like female, Kallmann syndrome can affect men leading to hypogonadotropic hypogonadism. Given, the X-linked recessive and sometimes autosomal dominant and recessive mode of transmission, men with it should receive genetic screening, as recommended by European Urology Association (EUA).[23] This can estimate the risk of transmission to the offspring, although very few laboratories can do such testing.[23] In men with Kallmann syndrome, the spermatogenesis can be easily induced by hormonal treatment like pulsatile GnRH therapy or gonadotrophins [human chorionic gonadotropin (hCG) with or without FSH].[23] However, initiation of spermatogenesis can take 6–24 months of time in some cases.[23] Given ease of administration and cost, gonadotrophin is preferred to pulsatile GnRH therapy. In most cases natural conception is possible after hormone therapy, even when the sperm parameters are subnormal.[23] Therefore, these men often do not need assisted reproductive techniques.

Obstructive Azoospermia

Congenital bilateral absence of vas deferens (CBAVD) is associated with obstructive azoospermia (OA) and can be associated with cystic fibrosis (CF).[23] The incidence varies depending on the ethnicity.[23] In the Caucasian, the CF is the most common genetic defect, often caused by the mutation of the gene, CF transmembrane conductance regulator (CFTR), which controls the ion channels.[23] This gene, located on the chromosome number 7, controls the influences, the development of the Wolffian ducts, particularly, the ejaculatory ducts, seminal vesicles, vas deferens, and part of the epididymis and therefore, it is not surprising why CFTR mutation leads to OA.[23]

Because CBAVD may be the reason for OA, in men with azoospermia with semen volume <1.5 mL and pH <7.0, careful examination of vasa is needed, because clinically often the diagnosis of CBAVD can be missed.[23]

There are number of *CFTR* gene mutations, most common being F508. Routine testing can detect many, but not all of the mutations.[23] Men with CBAVD can show some stigmata of CF like recurrent chest infections.[23] because of the autosomal recessive pattern of transmission, if the genetic defect is detected in the male partner, the female partner should be tested before proceeding for ICSI.[23] If the female is the carrier, the risk of the baby being affected with CF is 50% whereas if the female partner is normal, the risk is 0.4% because of transmission of undetected mutations.[23]

Recommendations for Genetic Testing in Infertile Male

In all men with sperm concentration <10 million/mL, karyotype should be offered to diagnose sex chromosomal and sometimes autosomal defects.[23] Y chromosome microdeletion test should be offered in men with severe oligospermia and nonobstructive azoospermia. If AZFa or AZFb microdeletions are present, surgical sperm retrieval is discouraged.[23] *CFTR* gene mutation testing should be done in case of nonobstructive azoospermia because of CBAVD but all the mutations may not be detected by the commonly performed tests.[23] In addition men with unilateral absent vas and normal kidney should be offered this test.[23]

Other Roles of Genetics in Male Infertility

Because some infertility may be of genetic origin, infants born after ICSI may be at risk of carrying the same genetic abnormalities. Overall, there is increased chance of autosomal and sex chromosomal defects in men having severe problems in semen and by means of ICSI such defects can be transmitted to the offspring.[23] Therefore, the offspring may be at the risk of fertility problems. These abnormalities are usually detected by PGT. Men with karyotypic abnormalities, carriers of cystic fibrosis, and Y chromosome microdeletion should be offered PGT if ICSI is contemplated.[23]

Men with sperm defects are at risk of developing cardiovascular morbidities, diabetes, metabolic diseases, repeated hospitalization, and early mortality.[26,27] There are studies suggesting increased risk of cancer in infertile men and these include lymphoma, extragonadal germ cell tumors, peritoneal cancers, and testicular cancers.[23,26] The exact pathogenesis of testicular cancer in men with infertility is unclear.[26] Genetic mutations and chromosomal aneuploidies may be linked with such malignancies.[26] These include instability of Y-chromosome, abnormal Hiwi protein, and DNA mismatch repair. Another possible explanation is the "testicular dysgenesis syndrome" (TDS) which is characterized by abnormal semen parameters and urogenital abnormalities such as cryptorchidism, testicular germ cell tumor (TGCT), and hypospadias.[26] The pathogenesis of TDS starts probably from the embryonic life because of endocrine disruption mediated by the environmental factors and all these can increase the risk of both infertility and TGCT in TDS.[26] The EUA suggested teaching the testicular self-examination in men with testicular microlithiasis (TM) as a part of screening for testicular cancer.[23]

GENETICS FOR PREIMPLANTATION GENETIC TESTING

Preimplantation genetic testing is the technology to diagnose the genetic defects in the embryo and in this early genetic diagnostic test, only the embryos with no genetic defects are transferred into the uterine cavity.[28] Preimplantation genetic diagnosis (PGD) was developed from late 1980s as an alternative way to prenatal diagnosis for the couples who are at risk of transmitting genetic defects (such as cystic fibrosis) or chromosomal abnormalities (such as translocation) to their offspring.[28,29] The same technology was extended to the women with advanced age or RIF to screen the embryos for genetic defects, because it was then well established that genetically abnormal embryos were more likely to have failed implantation.[28,29] This was termed preimplantation genetic screening (PGS), developed by mid-1990s.[29] Later on PGS were applied to couples with severe male factor infertility and recurrent pregnancy loss (RPL).[28,30]

The term "PGT" has replaced both the previous terms PGD and PGS.[31] The newer terminologies are:
- PGT-A (PGT for aneuploidy)—previously called PGS
- PGT-SR (PGT for structural rearrangement of chromosomes)—previously under PGD
- PGT-M (PGT for Mendelian or single gene disorders)—previously under PGD.[31,32]

Recurrent Pregnancy Loss

Genetic assessment of pregnancy-tissue can be considered for testing by array-comparative genomic hybridization (a-CGH).[30] Parental karyotype may give information about possible contributory factor for RPL.[30] It can also provide information regarding prognosis in future pregnancy, because the chance of subsequent pregnancy loss is high.[30] The pregnancy loss depends on the type of chromosomal abnormalities, because the risk is higher in couples having unbalanced translocation, reciprocal translocations, and inversions than those with Robertsonian translocations. However, in couples with chromosomal abnormalities, only 1/3 of the pregnancy loss is caused solely by genetic factors. Other underlying factors still can be present.[30] Although the risk of subsequent miscarriage is high, the live birth rate is quite good (63%).[30] Moreover, conventional karyotyping does not exclude the possibility of having baby with unbalanced translocation.[30] Therefore, the European Society of Human Reproduction and Embryology (ESHRE) recommended parental karyotyping in selective cases after doing individual risk-assessment in the following cases:

- Previous baby with congenital anomalies
- Unbalanced translocation in offspring of any family members
- Translocation in the pregnancy tissue.[30]

Genetic counseling should be offered in cases of abnormalities in parental karyotypes.[30] Normally, the couple has the options such as (1) IVF with PGT-SR, (2) natural conception and PND (prenatal diagnosis), and (3) third party reproduction. The advantage of PGT is that it can reduce the risk of miscarriage.[30] However, PGT may not improve the live birth rate.[30] Additionally, there is chance, especially at the age of 44, when ovarian reserve is likely to be compromised, that no euploid blastocyst may be obtained for transfer.[30] There is insufficient evidence to suggest benefits of PGT in couples with RPL and therefore, further robust quality of studies is required.[30]

Recurrent Implantation Failure

First of all, it should be emphasized that although embryo aneuploidy may play major role in RIF, the endometrial factors should not be underestimated. The structural and infective pathologies may also be responsible for repeated failure.[33-35]

Secondly, there have been changes in the terminology. If any one of the partners is found to carry balanced translocation, there is high risk of embryo aneuploidy.[34] Therefore, karyotyping should be offered in all the couples with RIF.[35] Those found to carry structural rearrangement like balanced translocation, should be offered PGT-SR.[35] On the other hand, women aged >40 years are often producing embryos with aneuploidy despite the fact that both the partner may carry normal karytypes.[25,34] Therefore, selection of the best quality of embryo in this case can be done by PGT-A.[35,36] However, the evidences are showing controversial results regarding the benefits of PGT-A.[35] It is important to note that, even if any person opts for PGT-A, the ideal biopsy can be obtained from trophoectoderm of a blastocyst, rather than from blastomere of day 3 embryo.[36] The former has many advantages like more accurate, more informative, and is associated with more live birth rate.[35]

CONCLUSION

Advanced exome and genome sequencing, phenotyping helped a lot to unreveal genetic causes of different factors like genital tract developmental defects, primary ovarian insufficiencies, recurrent pregnancy losses etc. Polygenic nature of postfertilization embryo developmental failure can also direct future research to go into more depth for better management of infertile couples.

REFERENCES

1. Jacquinet A, Millar D, Lehman A. Etiologies of uterine malformations. Am J Med Genet. 2016;170:2141-72.
2. Tuke MA, Ruth KS, Wood AR, Beaumont RN, Tyrrell J, Jones SE, et al. Mosaic Turner syndrome shows reduced penetrance in an adult population study. Genet Med. 2019;21:877-86.
3. Abir R, Fisch B, Nahum R, Orvieto R, Nitke S, Ben Rafael Z. Turner's syndrome and fertility: current status and possible putative prospects. Hum Reprod Update. 2001;7(6):603-10.
4. Lakhal B, Braham R, Berguigua R, Bouali N, Zaouali M, Chaieb M, et al. Cytogenetic analyses of premature ovarian failure using karyotyping and interphase fluorescence in situ hybridization (FISH) in a group of 1000 patients. Clin Genet. 2010;78:181-5.
5. Stochholm K, Juul S, Juel K, Naeraa RW, Gravholt CH. Prevalence, incidence, diagnostic delay, and mortality in Turner syndrome. J Clin Endocrinol Metabol. 2006; 91(10):3897-02.
6. Hadnott TN, Gould HN, Gharib AM, Bondy CA. Outcomes of spontaneous and assisted pregnancies in Turner syndrome: the U.S. National Institutes of Health experience. Fertil Steril. 2011;95(7):2251-22.
7. Eggers S, Ohnesorg T, Sinclair A. Genetic regulation of mammalian gonad development. Nat Rev Endocrinol. 2014;11:673-83.
8. Ono M, Harley VR. Disorders of sex development: new genes, new concepts. Nat Rev Endocrinol. 2013;2:79-91.
9. King TF, Conway GS. Swyer syndrome. Curr Opin Endocrinol Diabetes Obes. 2014;6:504-10.
10. Tsutsumi M, Fujiwara R, Nishizawa H, Ito M, Kogo H, Inagaki H, et al. Age-related decrease of meiotic cohesins in human oocytes. PLoS One. 2014;9:e96710.
11. Wood-Trageser MA, Gurbuz F, Yatsenko SA, Jeffries EP, Kotan LD, Surti U, et al. MCM9 mutations are associated with ovarian failure, short stature, and chromosomal instability. Am J Hum Genet. 2014;95:754-62.
12. AlAsiri S, Basit S, Wood-Trageser MA, Yatsenko SA, Jeffries EP, Surti U, et al. Exome sequencing reveals MCM8 mutation underlies ovarian failure and chromosomal instability. J Clin Invest. 2015;125:258-62.
13. Tenenbaum-Rakover Y, Weinberg-Shukron A, Renbaum P, Lobel O, Eideh H, Gulsuner S, et al. Minichromosome

maintenance complex component 8 (MCM8) gene mutations result in primary gonadal failure. J Med Genet. 2015;52:391-9.
14. Conti M, Franciosi F. Acquisition of oocyte competence to develop as an embryo: integrated nuclear and cytoplasmic events. Hum Reprod Update. 2018;24:245-66.
15. Jiang M, Aittomäki K, Nilsson C, Pakarinen P, Iitiä A, Torresani T, et al. The frequency of an inactivating point mutation (566C→T) of the human follicle-stimulating hormone receptor gene in four populations using allele-specific hybridization and time-resolved fluorometry. J Clin Endocrinol Metab. 1998;83:4338-43.
16. Siegel ET, Kim HG, Nishimoto HK, Layman LC. The molecular basis of impaired Follicle-Stimulating hormone action. Reprod Sci. 2013;20:211-33.
17. Garcia-Cruz R, Brieno MA, Roig I, Grossmann M, Velilla E, Pujol A, et al. Dynamics of cohesin proteins REC8, STAG3, SMC1 beta and SMC3 are consistent with a role in sister chromatid cohesion during meiosis in human oocytes. Hum Reprod. 2010;25:2316-27.
18. Sanfins A, Rodrigues P, Albertini DF. GDF-9 and BMP-15 direct the follicle symphony. J Assist Reprod Genet. 2018;35:1741-50.
19. Huang L, Tong X, Wang F, Luo L, Jin R, Fu Y, et al. Novel mutations in PATL2 cause female infertility with oocyte germinal vesicle arrest. Hum Reprod. 2018;33:1183-90.
20. Khastgir G, Abdalla H, Thomas A, Korea L, Latarche L, Studd J. Oocyte donation in Turner's syndrome: an analysis of the factors affecting the outcome. Hum Reprod. 1997;12(2):279-85.
21. Borgstrom B, Hreinsson J, Rasmussen C, Sheikhi M, Fried G, Keros V, et al. Fertility preservation in girls with turner syndrome: prognostic signs of the presence of ovarian follicles. J Clin Endocrinol Metabol. 2009;94(1): 74-80.
22. Balen AH, Harris SE, Chambers EL, Picton HM. Conservation of fertility and oocyte genetics in a young woman with mosaic Turner syndrome. BJOG. 2010;117(2):238-42.
23. Jungwirth A, Diemer T, Kopa Z, Krausz C, Minhas S, Tournaye H. EAU Guidelines on male infertility. European Association of Urology. 2018.
24. Hawksworth DJ, Szafran AA, Jordan PW, Dob AS, Herati AS. Infertility in patients with Klinefelter syndrome: optimal timing for sperm and testicular tissue cryopreservation. 2018 Rev Urol. 2018;20(2):56-62.
25. Corona G, Pizzocaro A, Lanfranco F, Garolla A, Pelliccione F, Vignozzi L, et al. Sperm recovery and ICSI outcomes in Klinefelter syndrome: a systematic review and meta-analysis. Hum Reprod Update. 2017;23(3): 265-75.
26. Choy JT, Eisenberg ML. Comprehensive men's health and male infertility. Transl Androl Urol. 2020;9(Suppl 2): S239-43.
27. Bungum AB, Glazer CH, Bonde JP, Nilsson PM, Giwercman A, Søgaard Tøttenborg S. Risk of metabolic disorders in childless men: a population-based cohort study. BMJ Open. 2018;8(8):e020293.
28. Parikh FR, Athalye AS, Naik NJ, Naik DJ, Sanap RR, Madon PF. Preimplantation genetic testing: its evolution, where are we today? J Hum Reprod Sci. 2018;11(4): 306-14.
29. Harper JC. Preimplantation genetic screening. J Med Screen. 2018;25(1):1-5.
30. ESHRE Guideline Group on RPL, Bender Atik R, Christiansen OB, Elson J, Kolte AM, Lewis S, et al. ESHRE guideline: recurrent pregnancy loss. Hum Reprod Open. 2018(2);hoy004.
31. Zegers-Hochschild F, Adamson GD, Dyer S, Racosky C, de Mouzon J, Sokol R, et al. The International Glossary on Infertility and Fertility Care, 2017. Fertil Steril. 2017; 108:393-406.
32. Sciorio R, Tramontano L, Catt J. Preimplantation genetic diagnosis (PGD) and genetic testing for aneuploidy (PGT-A): status and future challenges. Gynecol Endocrinol. 2020;36(1):6-11.
33. Shahine LK, Marshall L, Lamb JD, Hickok LR. Higher rates of aneuploidy in blastocysts and higher risk of no embryo transfer in recurrent pregnancy loss patients with diminished ovarian reserve undergoing in vitro fertilization. Fertil Steril. 2016;106:1124-8.
34. Bashiri A, Halper KI, Orvieto R. Recurrent implantation failure-update overview on etiology, diagnosis, treatment and future directions. Reprod Biol Endocrinol. 2018; 16(1):121.
35. Reichman D, Kang HJ, Rosenwaks Z. Analysis of fertilization. In: Gardner DK, Weissman A, Howles CM, Shoham Z (Eds). Textbook of Assisted Reproductive Techniques. 5th edition. Florida: Taylor and Francis Group. 2018. pp: 662-73.
36. Lewin J, Wells D. Preimplantation genetic diagnosis for infertility. In: Gardner DK, Weissman A, Howles CM, Shoham Z (Eds). Textbook of Assisted Reproductive Techniques. 5th edition. Florida: Taylor and Francis Group. 2018. pp 350-8.

Chapter 10

Genetics and Recurrent Pregnancy Loss

Debasmita Mandal, Jyotshna Rani Panigrahi

INTRODUCTION

Although miscarriage is common, occurring in 15–25% of all clinically recognized pregnancies, recurrent pregnancy loss (RPL), defined as the loss of two or more clinical pregnancies, is uncommon. Among them 5% of women will experience two consecutive losses, and only 1% will experience three or more.[1] RPL is often idiopathic. Of the 50% of cases that have a discernible causes. While fetal chromosomal abnormalities are responsible for 70% of sporadic miscarriages, they account for considerably smaller fraction of pregnancy losses in RPL couples. Genetic causes are responsible for usually early pregnancy loss.

The couples with RPL can be divided into subgroups according to their reproductive history: primary (no successful pregnancies), secondary (series of miscarriages after a live birth) and tertiary (three nonconsecutive miscarriages) RPL and they should be considered as separate entities representing probably different pathophysiological mechanisms leading to pregnancy loss.[2]

This review will focus on genetic associations of RPL.

ANEUPLOIDY

Numerous chromosomal abnormalities can cause pregnancy loss. These are meiotic nondisjunction (e.g., trisomy or monosomy), aberrant fertilization (e.g., triploidy), or embryogenesis (e.g., tetraploidy), or because of structural chromosomal abnormalities, arising from the inheritance of a derivative chromosome (e.g., translocations and inversions).[1] Incidence and outcome of various karyotypic abnormalities are shown in **Table 1**.[1]

Ndamkou et al. had studied the age-related risk of recurrent miscarriages as J-shaped, with an outcome of lowest risk (9.8%) among women aged 25–29 years.[3]

TABLE 1: Estimated incidence and outcome of various karyotypic abnormalities in 10,000 pregnancies.

	Incidence per 10,000 pregnancies	Spontaneous abortion (%)	Live births
Total	10,000	1,500 (15)	8,500
Normal chromosomes	9,200	750 (8)	8,450
Abnormal chromosomes	800	750 (94)	50
Specific abnormalities			
Polyploid	170	170 (100)	0
45,X	140	139 (99)	1
Trisomy 16	112	112 (100)	0
Trisomy 18	20	19 (95)	1
Trisomy 21	45	35 (78)	10
Trisomy, other	209	208 (99.5)	1
47, XXY; 47, XXX; 47, XYY	19	4 (21)	15
Unbalanced rearrangement	27	23 (85)	4
Balanced rearrangement	19	3 (16)	16
Other	39	37 (95)	2

Recurrent losses in pregnancy loss rise in women aged 30–35 years to 33.2% in women aged 40–44 years and almost 50% in women over the age. Mainly chromosome errors (aneuploidy) in the conceptus, with meiosis faults accounting for >90% of aneuploidy when abortions are related to age. That is why the incidence of age-related meiotic errors in preimplantation embryos and oocytes simulates as the J-shaped curve in the age-related pregnancy loss risk (**Fig. 1**). Another risk factor remains is previous number of pregnancy losses.

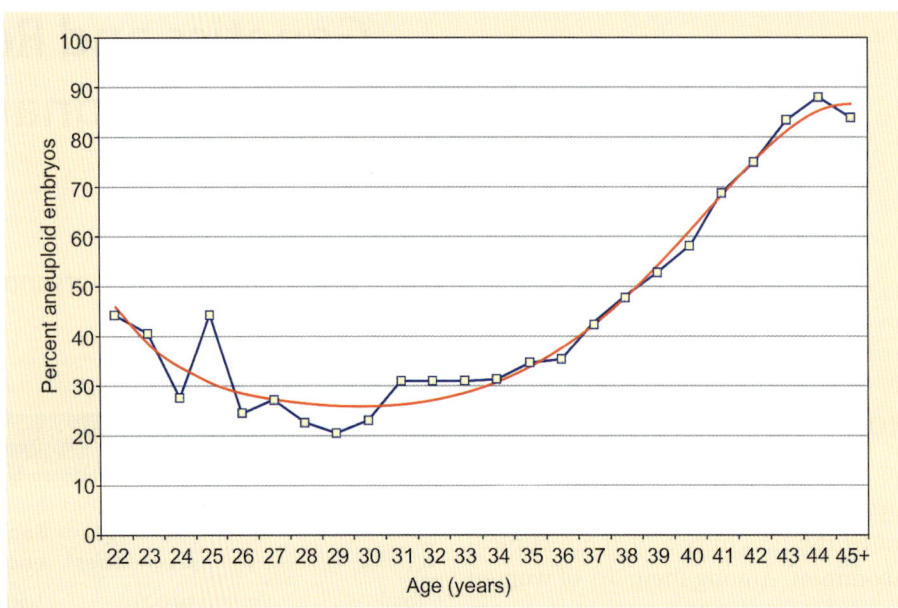

Fig. 1: Relativeness of prevalence of embryonic aneuploidy to female age in a general infertility population.[1]

■ TRANSLOCATION

Chromosomal translocation is defined as the interchange of genetic materials between two nonhomologous chromosomes. Pregnancy loss cases suggested that 1.3% harbors an unbalanced translocation in the fetus, with potential being inherited from balanced carrier parent. Approximately 2–5% of couples with RPL have been estimated to have a balanced reciprocal translocation.[4] Carriers of a balanced translocation may usually be phenotypically normal; their pregnancies are at greater risk of RPL or may result in a live birth with multiple congenital malformations and/or intellectual disability secondary to a balanced chromosomal arrangement **(Figs. 2A to F)**. It is highly recommended to those couples in whom one partner is at risk of harboring a chromosomal translocation screening.

■ COPY NUMBER VARIATIONS

Most copy number variations (CNVs) associated with RPL have lengths ranging between 2 MB and 400 kB. The most common region of pathogenic CNVs was the highly imprinted region 11p15.5. This region is abundant with imprinted genes and has a vital role in the maternal-fetal exchange.[5] Aberrant methylation or duplication of imprinted genes in this region could cause RPL. Recurrent CNVs have been found to be associated with RPL. A large cohort of >7,000 samples of placenta has been examined by array comparative genomic hybridization (CGH), and the team discovered chromosomal aneuploidy in 53% of the loss; besides, submicroscopic abnormalities, including deletions, duplications, multiple regions of homozygosity, and variants of uncertain significance, were associated with another 5.08% of the PL.

■ MOSAICISM

Confined placental mosaicism (CPM) is the chromosomal differences between the fetus and placenta. Literature reviewed that roughly 10% of trisomic conceptions contained a mosaic cell line.[6] Even this mosaicism was shown to be associated with an increased possibility of second- and third-trimester RPL and intrauterine fetal growth retardation. Over the entire gestational period, CPM can be found in over 2% of viable pregnancies. Aneuploidy in a fetus may affect organ function, and placental aneuploidy also frequently leads to malfunction, resulting in growth retardation or even death from placental insufficiency. Chromosomal microarray (CMA) and whole exome sequencing (WES) both are better in predicting the mosaics.

■ MUTATIONS AND SINGLE NUCLEIC VARIATIONS

Several inborn metabolic errors, hemoglobinopathies, and X-linked disorders are associated with RPL.[4]

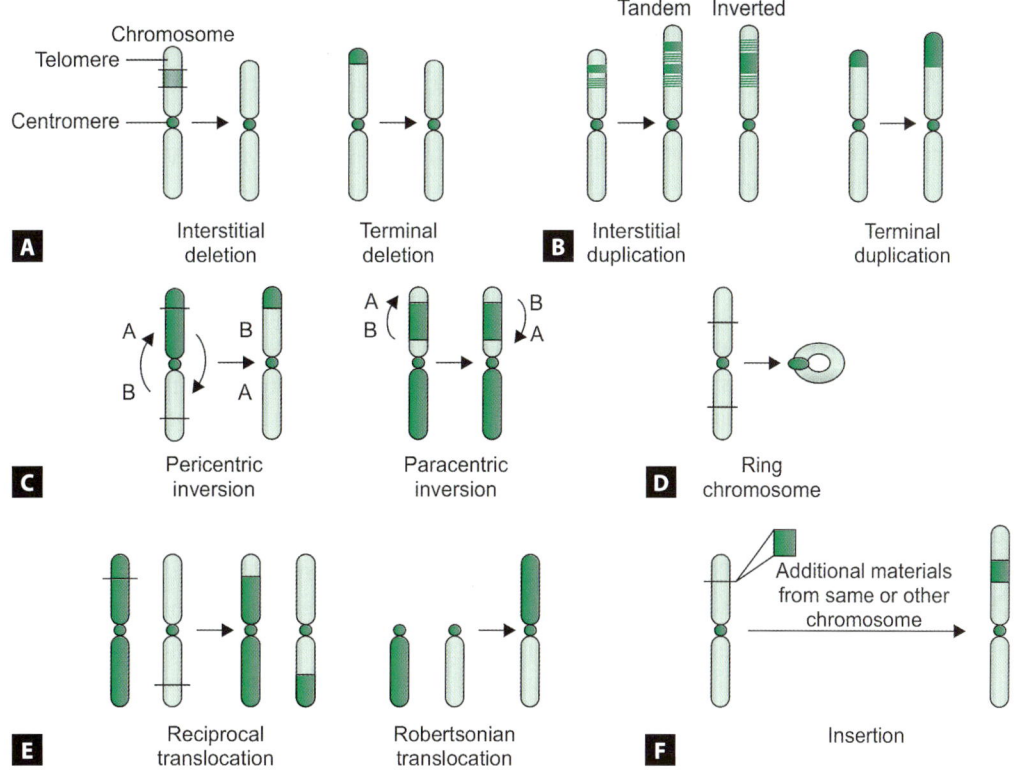

Figs. 2A to F: Pictures of anatomical chromosomal rearrangements; (A) deletions; (B) duplications; (C) ring chromosome; (D) isochromosomes; (E) Robertsonian translocations; (F) reciprocal translocations.[1]

Severe untreated α-thalassemia may lead to universal fetal loss.[7] Most of the mutations or single nucleotide polymorphisms (SNPs) found in aborted fetuses were inherited from one or both side(s) of the parents. One team examined a family with RPL due to nonimmune hydrops fetalis by exome sequencing and identified a novel missense mutation in CHRNA1 responsible for this medical condition.[8] The same group studied 24 consanguineous families with RPL due to lethal nonimmune hydrops fetalis and then scree them with exome sequencing and pathogenic homozygous mutations were identified in seven genes.[9] Recurrent mutations in this cohort were detected in one of the genes (THSD1) with a role in angiogenesis and maintenance of vascular integrity.[10] In 2018, the team studied 44 more families with lethal pregnancy outcomes and pathogenic variants were observed in 50% of these families.

■ EPIGENETIC STUDIES

Epigenetic factors are important for maintaining correct gene expression to ensure cellular and tissue homeostasis, especially during various reproduction processes, including meiosis, embryo development, implantation, tissue remodeling, and pregnancy maintenance. Dysregulation in epigenetic mechanisms may lead to disturbances in the normal biological process and result in many diseases, such as uncertain RPL.[4]

Among the different alterations, the unbalanced inactivation of maternal and paternal X chromosomes in women [also known as skewed X chromosome inactivation (SXCI)] has been associated with RPL. Somatic cells from female mammals contain two X chromosomes, one of which is randomly inactivated during the embryonic period, resulting in one functional X chromosome in all cells throughout life.[11] In normal females, the inactivation occurs randomly so that each X chromosome (maternal or paternal) remains active in approximately 50% of somatic cells.

A study based on Mexican couples with three or more losses identified heterochromatin polymorphism in 29.1% of the male member and 21.5% of the female member of the couples.[12]

Polymorphisms of rs12976445 and rs41275794 in pri-miR-125a alter mature miRNA expression and associate with RPL in the Chinese population.[12] Functional investigation illustrated that mutant pri-miR-125a can disturb the expression of miR-125a targetome and then enhance the invasive capacity of endometrial stromal cells.

EVALUATION OF PRODUCTS OF CONCEPTION

Various advantages are with SNP microarray or array CGH. Because cell culture is not required as well as a shorter time spent in whole process. High resolution provides detection of microduplications and microdeletions below the traditional 10-Mb resolution of G-banding.

MANAGEMENT OPTIONS FOR GENETIC ISSUES OF RECURRENT PREGNANCY LOSS

Individualized approach to RPL is the best way out for management **Flowchart 1**. For couples with recurrent aneuploidy or unbalanced losses, the available options include in vitro fertilization (IVF)/preimplantation genetic screening (PGS)/preimplantation genetic diagnosis (PGD). The ideal study would randomize patients with RPL (two clinical losses with sonographic or pathologic confirmation) to EM or IVF with blastocyst biopsy **(Fig. 3)**, molecular analysis using a contemporary PGS platform and planned frozen embryo transfer.[1]

CONCLUSION

In summary, the etiopathogenetic of RPL is complex and often multifactorial with genetic factors involving not only abnormal karyotypes but also chromosomal polymorphisms. It needs good studies from different geographical locations. Simultaneously, we should consider good genetic counseling and pregnancy screening in RPL prediction. In clinical practice, physicians should take a detailed medical history, and some ancillary tests to rule out other causes except genetic also. Patients with RPL should be monitored more closely during pregnancy and should be managed at tertiary care center.

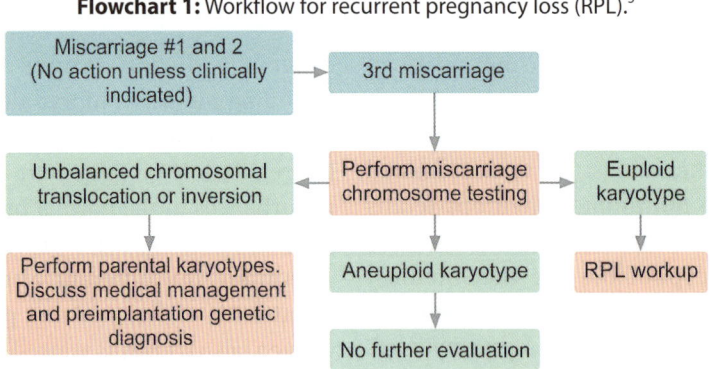

Flowchart 1: Workflow for recurrent pregnancy loss (RPL).[3]

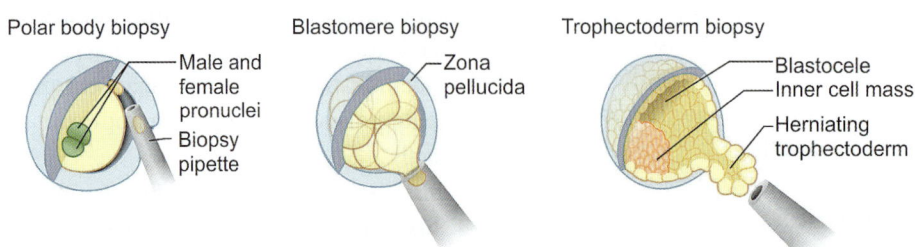

Fig. 3: Biopsy methods for preimplantation genetic analysis.[13]

REFERENCES

1. Kaser D. The status of genetic screening in recurrent pregnancy loss. Obstet Gynecol Clin N Am. 2018;45:143-54.
2. Rull K, Nagirnaja L, Laan M. Genetics of recurrent miscarriage: challenges, current knowledge, future directions. Front Genet. 2012;3:34.
3. Ndjapa-Ndamkou C, Govender L, Chauke L. Role of genetic factors in recurrent miscarriages—A review. Afr J Reprod Health. 2022;26(10):72-82.
4. Zhao X, Zhong N. Genetic studies of pregnancy loss. Am J Biomed Sci Res. 2021;12(5).
5. Zhang H, Liu W, Chen M, Li Z, Sun X, Wang C. Implementation of a high-resolution single-nucleotide polymorphism array in analyzing the products of conception. Genet Test Mol Biomarkers. 2016;20(7):352-8.
6. Kalousek DK. Confined placental mosaicism and intrauterine development. Pediatr Pathol. 1990;10(1-2):69-77.
7. Kalousek DK, Barrett IJ, Gärtner AB. Spontaneous abortion and confined chromosomal mosaicism. Hum Genet. 1992;88(6):642-6.
8. Origa R, Moi P. Alpha-Thalassemia. In: Adam MP, Mirzaa GM, Pagon RA, Wallace SE, Bean LJH, Gripp KW, et al. (Eds.). GeneReviews. Seattle (WA), USA; 1993.
9. Shamseldin HE, Swaid A, Alkuraya FS. Lifting the lid on unborn lethal Mendelian phenotypes through exome sequencing. Genet Med. 2013;15(4):307-9.
10. Shamseldin HE, Tulbah M, Kurdi W, Nemer M, Alsahan N, Al Mardawi E, et al. Identification of embryonic lethal genes in humans by autozygosity mapping and exome sequencing in consanguineous families. Genome Biol. 2015;16(1):116.
11. Lyon MF. Sex chromatin and gene action in the mammalian X-chromosome. Am J Hum Genet. 1962;14:135-48.
12. De la Fuente-Cortés BE, Cerda-Flores RM, Dávila-Rodríguez MI, García-Vielma C, De la Rosa Alvarado RM, Cortés-Gutiérrez EI. Chromosomal abnormalities and polymorphic variants in couples with repeated miscarriage in Mexico. Reprod Biomed Online. 2009;18(4):543-8.
13. Hu Y, Liu CM, Qi L, He TZ, Shi-Guo L, Hao CJ, et al. Two common SNPs in pri-miR-125a alter the mature miRNA expression and associate with recurrent pregnancy loss in a Han-Chinese population. RNA Biol. 2011;8(5):861-72.

Preimplantation Genetic Diagnosis

11 Chapter

Dipanjana Datta

■ INTRODUCTION

Preimplantation genetic testing (PGT)/preimplantation genetic diagnosis/preimplantation genetic screening is a process where embryos can be screened after fertilization for genetic conditions or for social sex selection in foreign countries and a healthy/chosen embryo can be used for implantation. PGT is an important accessory to assisted reproductive technologies (ART), since it can lower the risk of later elective pregnancy termination for reasons of debilitating inherited genetic condition/increase the chance of live births by screening chromosomal imbalances.[1]

■ HISTORY

Two significant breakthroughs made the process of PGT possible. The first discovery was the ability to maintain an embryo in a laboratory for up to 8 days. The second discovery was the development of advanced molecular testing that was sensitive. These advancements in the technology of in vitro fertilization (IVF) paved the way for further progress. In 1988, Marilyn Monk, along with Audrey Muggleton-Harris from the UK, developed the trophectoderm biopsy technique and PGT using biochemical microarray in a mouse model for Lesch-Nyhan disease. At the same time, Yury Verlinsky's group reported the presence of a maternal unaffected gene by the first polar body biopsy. Successful implementation of these techniques in the mouse model was crucial for Alan Handyside and his team, who reported pregnancies performing PGT for sex-linked disease and X-linked mental retardation on biopsied human preimplantation embryos. They were able to identify male, female, and Turner syndrome embryos. Verlinsky et al. reported the first successful PGT with human leukocyte antigen matching for a sibling with Fanconi anemia by haplotype analysis.[2]

PROCESS DEVELOPMENT AND TESTING PLATFORMS FOR PREIMPLANTATION GENETIC TESTING

Despite advances, PGT was not widely used. In 2007, Mastenbroek's group conducted a multicentric, randomized controlled trial (RCT) in women aged 35–41 years who underwent IVF for three cycles with PGT. They used fluorescent in situ hybridization (FISH) as the molecular method to screen embryos. The trial showed that birth rates were 10% lower in women who underwent PGT compared to those who did not undergo it. This negative publication led to reduced use of PGT for the next few years. However, Munne and other scientists later highlighted the concept of better pregnancy outcomes using PGT. By this time, the art of embryo biopsy had been perfected and more sensitive and specific molecular genetic testing methods such as array comparative genome hybridization (aCGH) had been developed. Different groups around the world reported that cleavage-stage biopsy on day 5 was better than blastocyst biopsy on day 3 for embryo implantation and live birth outcomes. Scott et al. indicated that biopsy of the cleavage-stage embryo had an aberrant implantation potential, while Capalbo et al. reported that trophectoderm biopsy on day 5/6 or blastocyst stage embryos improved outcomes. Meta-analysis by Dahdouh et al. of various RCT and observational studies showed that PGT performed with comprehensive chromosome screening (CCS) improved clinical implantation rate (IR) and sustained IR (beyond 20 weeks) compared to routine methods of embryo selection in IVF cycles. After 2010, the introduction of more sophisticated molecular methods for CCS, such as single-nucleotide polymorphism (SNP) testing, quantitative real-time polymerase chain reaction (QT-PCR), and next-generation sequencing (NGS), further improved outcomes and reduced time. Around the same time, the concept of euploid single embryo transfer (eSET) was introduced. Forman et al. compared CCS-eSET group with non-CCS with SET group and showed higher ongoing pregnancy rates and lower miscarriage rates in CCS-eSET group. The implementation of embryos undergoing NGS-based PGT-A revealed higher implantation rates and live birth rates than those with aCGH, which might be attributed to the advantages of NGS in detecting microdeletions, microduplications, and mosaicism.[2]

INDICATIONS FOR PREIMPLANTATION GENETIC TESTING

The current indications for PGT include repeated implantation failures (RIF), repeated pregnancy loss (RPL), advanced maternal and paternal age (RMA/RPA), male factor infertility (MF), and inherited genetic disorders in the family including mosaicism of sex chromosomes, structural rearrangements, and monogenic genetic diseases.

Preimplantation genetic testing according to the requirement is divided into the following subtypes.

Preimplantation Genetic Testing for Aneuploidy

Embryonic chromosomal aneuploidy is responsible for around 70% of spontaneous miscarriages. Women undergoing IVF, regardless of age, have been found to have aneuploidy in their embryos. Preimplantation genetic testing for aneuploidy [PGT (A)] is a screening process that detects numerical aneuploidy. PGT (A) is recommended in cases of recurrent implantation failure, advanced maternal age, male factor infertility (unexplained severe teratozoospermia), and recurrent miscarriage due to a genetic condition. NGS technology has identified mosaicism and sub-chromosomal variations, including segmental aneuploidies, which were previously undetected. Implementing NGS-based PGT-A on embryos has resulted in higher implantation rates (71.6% of 548 cycles vs. 64.6% of 368 cycles) and live birth rates (LBRs) (62% vs. 54.4%) than aCGH. The advantages of NGS include its ability to detect microdeletions, microduplications, and mosaicism.[2]

Preimplantation Genetic Testing for Structural Rearrangements

Structural chromosomal rearrangements (SRs) can take on the form of segmental aneuploidy, which results in the presence of extra or missing parts of chromosomes when unbalanced. When balanced, SRs are generally asymptomatic and only identified when an individual attempts to conceive. Carriers of balanced SRs may experience infertility or subfertility, repeated miscarriage, and recurrent stillbirth, along with fetal or infant congenital disorders. The fertility phenotype may also be influenced by factors such as the type of rearrangement (balanced translocation, Robertsonian translocation, inversion, etc.), chromosomal breakage points, and the presence of an interchromosomal effect (ICE). In cases such as these, PGT-SR may be offered as an alternative to prenatal diagnosis. Different sampling approaches and genomic analysis techniques have been used to isolate normal (or balanced SR) embryos. PGT-SR techniques have benefited greatly from the advances made in PGT. Huang et al. reported significant success in patients carrying reciprocal translocations with PGT-SR. Prior to PGT-SR treatment, 83.8% of 592 pregnancies resulted in miscarriage, 13.3% had induced labor or congenital disabilities, and only 2.9% resulted in normal newborns. After undergoing PGT-SR, clinical pregnancies occurred, with 85.6% resulting in normal live births. Although not all miscarriages or birth defects were prevented, PGT-SR demonstrated an improvement in pregnancy outcomes.[2]

Preimplantation Genetic Testing for Monogenic Disorders

Monogenic disorders can be caused by pathogenic variations in a single gene. While these types of diseases are typically rare, the overall incidence rate exceeds 1%, and they can cause significant clinical issues such as intellectual or physical disabilities and in some cases even death. To prevent congenital disabilities caused by monogenic diseases before embryo transfer, preimplantation genetic testing for monogenic disorders (PGT-M) is crucial. Indications for PGT-M include X-linked disorders (such as Duchenne's muscular dystrophy), dominant single-gene disorders (like Huntington's disease), recessive single-gene disorders (such as cystic fibrosis), mitochondrial disorders (like Kearns–Sayre syndrome), human leukocyte antigen (HLA) typing (for "savior siblings"), and some severe disorders with high genetic predisposition (such as hereditary breast and ovarian cancer). However, it is important to highlight that PGT-M should only be used when the mutated gene has a clear pathogenic or gene-linked marker within the family, and the severity of the disease and circumstances of family members must be carefully considered. For late-onset disorders such as

Huntington's disease, exclusion or nondisclosure testing may be necessary to avoid presymptomatic testing of the partner with a family history of the disease. Exclusion testing is preferred over PGT with nondisclosure of direct test results to the couple. It is important to note that PGT-M may not detect euploidy of all chromosomes in embryos when diagnosing target gene mutations. Embryos with no pathogenic genes after PGT-M detection may still transfer chromosomal aneuploidy to the uterus, leading to adverse pregnancy outcomes. As studies have shown, combining PGT-A and PGT-M can improve live birth rates (with a 61.22% vs. 43.98% LBR in 98 and 438 cycles, respectively).[2]

Preimplantation Genetic Testing for Human Leukocyte Antigen

Preimplantation genetic testing for human leukocyte antigen (PGT-HLA only) is a process that involves the typing of human leukocyte antigen in a small number of cells extracted from in vitro fertilized preimplantation embryos. Its purpose is to establish a pregnancy that results in an HLA-compatible fetus, capable of undergoing hematopoietic stem cell transplantation (HSCT) to treat an affected sibling in need. PGT-M-HLA involves the identification of a compatible embryo, as well as detecting mutations responsible for immunodeficiencies and hemoglobinopathies. When considering exclusion from the process, factors such as the medical report of the affected child, prognosis, alternative treatments to PGT, and the results of previous HLA typing in affected child, parents, and siblings may be taken into account.[2]

Preimplantation Genetic Testing–MT

A strategy proposed by Spath et al. involves embryo biopsy and PGT to screen for both mitochondrial deoxyribonucleic acid (mtDNA) disease and aneuploidy simultaneously. This approach allows individuals at risk of transmitting mtDNA disease to maintain a biological connection with their offspring while ensuring the transfer of a euploid embryo free of mtDNA mutations. Previous studies have shown that mtDNA mutations associated with mtDNA disease often exhibit heteroplasmy, which means that wild-type and pathogenic mtDNA variants coexist within a single cell. The concept of heteroplasmy complicates mtDNA mutation inheritance because the proportion of pathogenic mtDNA inherited from one generation to the next varies widely due to a genetic bottleneck during oogenesis. Clinical symptoms occur only when the mutant load threshold exceeds a critical value. This phenomenon does not follow Mendelian genetics and may differ in penetrance by gender; thus, further validation of this technique is needed.[2]

Preimplantation Genetic Testing for Polygenic Disease Risk

Preimplantation genetic testing for polygenic disease risk (PGT-P) is a technique that involves examining each embryo through a biopsy, and then determining their polygenic risk based on genomic data. This allows for the selection of embryos with the lowest chance of developing polygenic disorders for implantation. The prevalence and impact of polygenic disorders, which are more common than monogenic disorders, makes PGT-P a necessary practice. Due to the complexity of polygenic conditions, the development of PGT-P was necessary. The polygenic score (PGS), which is calculated by adding up the weighted effect size of genotype based on genetic variations from genome-wide association study summary statistics, is the only approach that can estimate a person's genetic liability to a polygenic disorder at an individual level. Over the past few years, polygenic risk score (PRS) has accurately predicted multiple complex diseases, such as diabetes, cancers, cardiovascular diseases, and female reproductive system diseases, despite potential environmental influences.[2]

Noninvasive Preimplantation Genetic Testing

The first assessment of the potential for PGT using blastocyst fluid (BF)/spent blastocyst media to identify the sex of embryos was made by Palini et al. The development of NGS and the identification of DNA suitable for genetic testing and amplification in BF and spent culture medium (SCM) open a new chapter in noninvasive embryo viability testing (niEVT)/noninvasive preimplantation genetic testing (niPGT) technology. Without a doubt, eliminating embryo biopsy procedures would have benefits for both the economy and society. However, because there is not much cell-free DNA (cfDNA) in BF, there may occasionally be false positive or false negative results. More validation is required for this test.[2]

■ WHY IS IT A SCREENING TEST?

The PGT test is a screening test, which is used to identify few cells from the cytotrophoblast cells. It cannot detect all genetic abnormalities in a fetus, so prenatal counseling should be based on patients' individual risk factors, reproductive goals, and preferences. For example, a negative PGT result does not mean a baby without genetic abnormalities. False-positive and false-negative results can occur with the PGT test, so prenatal diagnostic testing [through chorionic villus sampling (CVS) or amniocentesis] should be offered to all patients who have achieved pregnancy after the PGT test. As PGT is used more often over time, data will be available to help determine the best prenatal testing and screening strategies for this population.

CONCLUSION

Primarily, advanced techniques have been introduced in PGT clinics and laboratory practices over time, leading to the use of PGT as a well-established accurate and safe procedure for addressing reproductive issues. The widespread implementation of genome-wide methods has enabled greater standardization and uniformity in PGT practices. As the cost of sequencing continues to decline, all-in-one PGT solutions, such as PGT Plus, are promising for clinic implementation. Other emerging PGT applications, such as niEVT/niPGT, though with ethical discussions and cannot completely replace conventional PGTs currently, do increase awareness among patients regarding the risks of transmitting genetic disorders to offspring. Together with the advances in people's living standards and declining testing costs, the global penetration of PGT services will continue to rise, and more people will benefit from PGT.

REFERENCES

1. Du R-Q, Zhao D-D, Kang K, Wang F, Xu R-X, Chi C-L, et al. A review of pre-implantation genetic testing technologies and applications. Reprod Dev Med. 2023;7(1):20-31.
2. Parikh FR, Athalye AS, Naik NJ, Naik DJ, Sanap RR, Madon PF. Preimplantation Genetic testing: its evolution, where are we today? J Human Reprod Sci. 2018;11(4): 306-14.

12 Genetics and Inherited Cancers

Saswati Mukhopadhyay

■ INTRODUCTION

Hereditary cancer syndromes (HCSs) are a heterogeneous group of genetic diseases, with significantly increased risk of tumor development. Cancer susceptibility is found in multiple syndromes such as Bloom syndrome, Fanconi anemia, Nijmegen breakage syndrome, ataxia-telangiectasia, etc. In most of these syndromes, there is biallelic inactivation of deoxyribonucleic acid (DNA) repair genes. The "genuine" HCSs, however, have no phenotypic malfunctions, only an increased risk of development of organ-specific malignant disease.

Genes involved in cancer are of two types—tumor suppressor genes and oncogenes.

1. *Oncogenes:* They are mutated copies of certain normal cellular genes called proto-oncogenes. Proto-oncogenes regulate normal cellular growth, division, and apoptosis. Oncogenes may lead to uncontrolled cell growth and the escape from cell death, which may result in cancer development.

    Examples: HER2, RAS, EGFR, etc.

2. Tumor-suppressor genes normally inhibit cell proliferation and tumor development. If mutated or deleted, these genes cannot function as negative regulators of cell proliferation allowing abnormal proliferation of tumor cells.

    Examples: p53, Rb, PTEN, BRCA1, BRCA2, etc.

■ MECHANISMS OF HEREDITARY CANCER PREDISPOSITION

Most of the HCS genes are tumor-suppressor genes, requiring biallelic inactivation to manifest as cancer. When inactivating pathogenic variant (PV) is inherited in a single allele, the remaining copy of the gene retains its function; thereby the normal health status is preserved. The process of malignant transformation is usually triggered by the "second hit", i.e., the remaining allele is inactivated by a somatic mutation. *RB1, BRCA1, BRCA2, MLH1, MSH2*—these HCS genes work in this way[1] **(Fig. 1)**.

Sometimes, mutated suppressor genes, in monoallelic form, may cause malignancy by reduced gene dosage (haploinsufficiency). A few cancers are caused by the inheritance of activated oncogene, e.g., multiple endocrine neoplasia (MEN) type 2A and 2B, associated with gain-of-function PVs in *RET* gene.

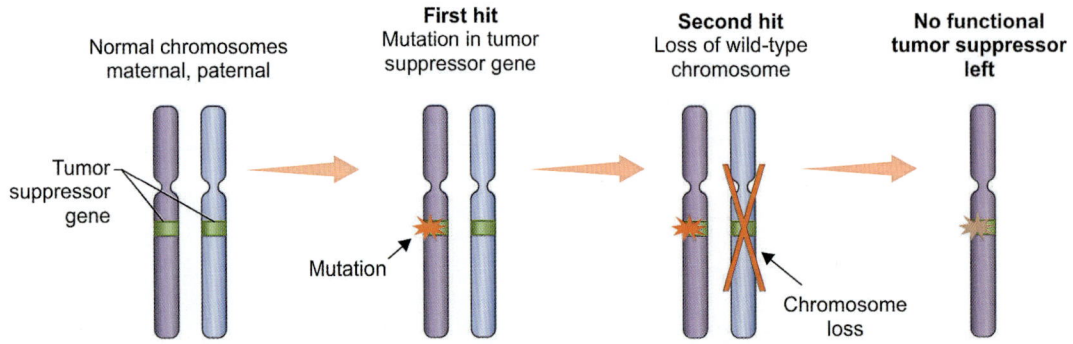

Fig. 1: Knudson's two-hit hypothesis for hereditary cancer syndrome (HCS).

MAJOR TYPES OF HEREDITARY CANCER SYNDROMES

Hereditary Breast and Ovarian Carcinomas

Families with a history of multiple breast or ovarian cancers approximately account for 15% of all patients with breast cancer.[2] Certain mutations in BRCA1 or 2 are responsible for most cases of hereditary breast and ovarian cancer (HBOC) syndrome. HBOC patients may also have an increased propensity for developing other types of cancer, such as melanoma, pancreatic, and prostate cancers. Hereditary breast cancer (BC) and hereditary ovarian cancer (OC) are represented by PVs located within the same genes, *BRCA1* and *BRCA2*, both of which are involved in double-strand DNA repair by homologous recombination. BC may also be a part of multiorgan cancer syndrome like Li–Fraumeni syndrome, diffuse stomach cancer. More than 2,900 variants of *BRCA1* and more than 3,400 variants of *BRCA2* pathogenic germline mutations are registered in ClinVar, a public archive of human genetic variants and interpretations of their significance to disease.[3]

BRCA1-related breast cancer has the following features:
- Histopathologically resembling medullary carcinoma
- High histological nuclear grade
- No expression of either estrogen and progesterone receptors or HER2 overexpression.

BRCA2-mutated breast cancer has the following features:
- Almost similar to those with *BRCA1* mutations
- Histologically high nuclear grade

High-grade serous adenocarcinoma has been found as a pathological feature of *BRCA1/2* ovarian cancer. Small cell carcinomas of the ovary, hypercalcemic type are related to germline PV in the *SMARCA4* gene, associated with chromatin remodeling.

Colorectal Cancer

Lynch syndrome, also called hereditary nonpolyposis colorectal cancer (HNPCC), is the most common genetic risk for colorectal cancer (CRC). Besides CRC, there is increased risk of endometrial cancer, gastric, small bowel, biliary, urothelial, ovarian, brain malignancies in Lynch syndrome.[4]

Some germline PVs predispose to polyposis of gastrointestinal tract; these polyps are commonly found to become malignant. Adenomatous polyposis coli (APC) is a tumor-suppressor gene, its inactivation results in upregulation of the WNT signaling pathway. APC is associated with highly increased risk of malignancy in the gastrointestinal (GI) tract. The incidence of APC is around 1:10,000.

Gastric Cancer

Gastric cancer (GC) risk is significantly increased when there is *Helicobacter pylori* infection, low hygienic standard, high consumption of salt, "Northern" diet, excessive alcohol intake. The role of heredity is obtained only for diffuse GC. This type of GC is poorly differentiated, with presence of signet-ring cells. The causative gene, *CDH1*, is associated with severely increased incidence of diffuse GC.[5] Other genes involved in GCs include *PALB2*, and the Lynch syndrome genes. The lifetime GC risk in carrier of *MLH1* or *MSH2* PVs is ~7–8%.

Other hereditary cancers include pancreatic cancer, prostate cancer, lung cancer, renal cancer, melanoma and the MEN1 and MEN2 syndromes **(Table 1)**.

Hereditary Cancer Syndromes

Li–Fraumeni syndrome: In the pediatric population, Li–Fraumeni syndrome is associated with adrenal cortical

TABLE 1: Genes involved with different types of hereditary cancers.

Malignancy	Genes involved
Breast and ovarian cancer	BRCA1, BRCA2, PALB2, ATM, and CHEK2, NBN (NBS1), BLM, RECQL, FANCM, BARD1
Ovarian cancer	ANKRD1, POLE, ERCC3, and SMARCA4
Lynch syndrome (HNPCC)	MLH1, MSH2, MSH6, PMS2, and EPCAM
Polyposis syndrome (polyposis in GIT)	APC, POLE, POLD1, STK11, SMAD4, BMPR1A, PTEN, GREM1, RNF43 (autosomal dominant) MUTYH, NTHL1, MSH3, and MBD4 (autosomal recessive)
Diffuse gastric cancer	CDH1
Renal cancer	VHL, FH, and FLCN
Lung cancer	EGFR
Prostate cancer	HOXB3, BRCA2, and ATM
Pancreatic cancer	PALB2 and BRCA2
Melanoma	CDKN2A, CDK4, POT1, and TERT

(HNPCC: hereditary nonpolyposis colorectal cancer)
Source: Imyanitov EN, Kuligina ES, Sokolenko AP, Suspitsin EN, Yanus GA, Iyevleva AG, et al. Hereditary cancer syndromes. World J Clin Oncol. 2023;14(2):40-68.

carcinomas, choroid plexus carcinomas, rhabdomyosarcomas, and medulloblastomas. In adults, Li–Fraumeni syndrome involves very young-onset BC in females, lung carcinomas, osteosarcomas, soft-tissue sarcomas, and brain tumors.

PTEN hamartoma tumor syndrome (Cowden syndrome): PTEN hamartoma tumor syndrome (PHTS) features multiple benign and malignant tumors of breast, thyroid, endometrium, skin, kidney, and colon.

Peutz–Jeghers syndrome (PJS): PJS is an autosomal dominant disease shows characteristic mucocutaneous pigmentations in the lips, eyes, nostrils, perianal area, mouth and of the buccal mucosa, and various polyps.

Multiple gastrointestinal hamartomatous polyps in the affected patients are located mainly in the small bowel, most commonly in jejunum and ileum. Stomach and colon polyps are also seen.

Gorlin syndrome: Gorlin syndrome, also called Gorlin-Goltz syndrome, basal cell nevus syndrome (BCNS), or nevoid basal cell carcinoma syndrome, is an autosomal dominant familial cancer syndrome. It is characterized by the appearance of BCCs and the development of odontogenic keratocysts. There is also increased risk of medulloblastoma.

Pediatric tumors: Retinoblastoma, Wilms' tumor (nephroblastoma), DICER1 syndrome

Hematological malignancies: Hereditary acute lymphoblastic leukemia, hereditary Hodgkin lymphoma.

The genes associated with hereditary cancer syndromes are listed in **Table 2**.

MANAGEMENT OF HEREDITARY TUMORS
Cancer Detection and Prevention

Female carriers of BRCA1, BRCA2:
- Breast self-examination, starting from 18 years of age
- Clinical breast examination annually
- Magnetic resonance imaging, starting from 25 years,
- Annual mammography between 30 and 75 years

Ovarian cancer screening:
- Transvaginal ultrasound examination annually to detect ovarian tumors
- CA-125 serum marker measurement yearly, starting at 30–35 years

TABLE 2: Genes involved with different types of hereditary cancers syndromes.

Syndromes	Genes
Li–Fraumeni syndrome	TP53
Multiple endocrine neoplasia (MEN) • MEN1—affects parathyroid glands, pancreatic islet cells and the anterior pituitary • MEN2—medullary thyroid carcinoma (MTC), pheochromocytoma • MEN3—highly metastatic and potentially fatal MTC, pheochromocytomas	MEN1 RET RET M918T allele, A883F allele
PTEN hamartoma tumor syndrome	PTEN
Peutz–Jeghers syndrome	STK11/LKB1 PVs
Gorlin syndrome	PTCH1, SUFU or PTCH2
Retinoblastoma	Rb
Neurofibromatosis	NF1
Wilms' tumor (nephroblastoma, WT)	WT1
DICER1 syndrome (pleuropulmonary blastomas, gynandroblastomas, sarcomas, Sertoli–Leydig cell tumors)	DICER1

Source: Imyanitov EN, Kuligina ES, Sokolenko AP, Suspitsin EN, Yanus GA, Iyevleva AG, et al. Hereditary cancer syndromes. World J Clin Oncol. 2023;14(2):40-68.

Patients with lynch syndrome:
- Colonoscopy should be performed every 1–2 years beginning from 20–25 years of age to detect suspicious ulcer
- Upper GI endoscopy every 3–5 years starting at 30–35 years
- Endometrial cancer screening by dilation and curettage (D&C) and endometrial sampling from 35 years, annually.

Carriers of highly-penetrant BC-predisposing pathogenic variants (*BRCA1, BRCA2, PALB2, TP53, etc.*) are encouraged to undergo:
- Mastectomy
- Prophylactic salpingo-oophorectomy at the age of 35–45 years (or after the completion of childbearing).

Advances in cytotoxic and targeted therapy: Several discoveries, made within the past 10–15 years have helped recognize specific drug vulnerabilities in hereditary cancers. Thus targeted therapies, aimed to the susceptible

TABLE 3: Cytotoxic and targeted therapy for tumors arising in carriers for cancer—predisposing alleles.

Tumor type	Target	Drugs
BRCA1/2-driven carcinomas	Deficiency of DNA repair by homologous recombination	Platinum derivatives, mitomycin C, bifunctional alkylating agents, PARPi
Microsatellite-unstable cancers, including tumors arising due to Lynch syndrome, POLE/POLD1, and MUTYH-related malignancies	Excessive number of somatic mutations and consequently, high tumor antigenicity	Immune checkpoint inhibitor—pembrolizumab
RET associated malignancies	RET tyrosine kinase	RET inhibitors—selpercatinib and pralsetinib
Neurofibromatosis, type 1	Upregulation of RAS/RAF/MEK pathway due to NF1 inactivation	MEK inhibitor—selumetinib
Gorlin syndrome	Hedgehog pathway	Smoothened (SMO) inhibitor—vismodegib
Tumors arising in patients with tuberous sclerosis	mTOR pathway	mTOR inhibitors
Renal cell carcinomas associated with Von Hippel–Lindau syndrome	Upregulation of HIF-2α due to VHL gene inactivation	HIF-2α inhibitor—belzutifan

(mTOR: mammalian target of rapamycin; PARPi: poly (ADP-ribose) polymerase inhibitor)
Source: Imyanitov EN, Kuligina ES, Sokolenko AP, Suspitsin EN, Yanus GA, Iyevleva AG, et al. Hereditary cancer syndromes. World J Clin Oncol. 2023;14(2):40-68.

pathways of the genetic mutations, are the new line of medical management of cancers[4] **(Table 3)**.

CONCLUSION

In those families in which multiple members have cancers in different/same target organs, genetic testing by whole exome or multigene sequencing should be offered to at-risk family members, after careful pretest counseling. Identifying the mutations in specific genes will help to screen at-risk family members, plan specific drug therapy for the patients and keep a strict vigilance on the target organs so that the cancer detection happens at the earliest stage. However, carrying the mutation does not mean developing the malignancy in the target organ, only the risk is increased, compared to the general population.

REFERENCES

1. Peltomäki P, Olkinuora A, Nieminen TT. Updates in the field of hereditary nonpolyposis colorectal cancer. Expert Rev Gastroenterol Hepatol. 2020;14:707-20.
2. Ford D, Easton DF, Bishop DT, Narod SA, Goldgar DE. Risks of cancer in BRCA1-mutation carriers. Breast Cancer Linkage Consortium. Lancet. 1994;343:692-5.
3. National Center for Biotechnology Information. ClinVar. [online] Available from: https://www.ncbi.nlm.nih.gov/clinv ar. [Last accessed October, 2023].
4. Imyanitov EN, Kuligina ES, Sokolenko AP, Suspitsin EN, Yanus GA, Iyevleva AG, et al. Hereditary cancer syndromes. World J Clin Oncol. 2023;14(2):40-68.
5. Guilford P, Hopkins J, Harraway J, McLeod M, McLeod N, Harawira P, et al. Ecadherin germline mutations in familial gastric cancer. Nature. 1998;392:402-5.

Gene Therapy

Shruti Jain, Meenakshi Lallar

■ INTRODUCTION

Gene therapy is the introduction of new genetic material into the cells. By this process either the new gene can be introduced or previous malfunctioning gene can be modified or replaced.[1] With recent advances, genome editing can also be done which induces precise cuts in genome and gene modification can be done. Theoretically as gene therapy aims to treat the genetic basis of disease rather than symptomatic treatment, it appears to be a more promising mode of treatment. Initially gene therapy was introduced as a cure for certain genetic disorders but it is slowly finding its application in cancers and multifactorial disorders as well.

Gene therapy seems to be the therapy of future wherein disorders that seem untreatable currently may have cure in future but it has lots of technical challenges and ethical challenges as well.

■ TYPES OF GENE THERAPY

As there are somatic and germline mutations, similarly there are two types of gene therapy:[2]
1. *Somatic gene therapy:* In this, gene therapy targets body cells and not gametes and hence is not passed to progeny. This is the therapy mostly used.
2. *Germline gene therapy:* In this, gene modification is done in gametes or fertilized eggs or early embryos. Modifications introduced through germline gene therapy are passed onto future generations. There are lots of concerns over safety, social, and ethical aspects of germline gene therapy. Germline gene therapy in healthy babies may lead to irreversible mutations that will be passed onto future generations making its safety questionable. There are ethical aspects about rights of unborn babies and therapy may be used to create designer babies. This therapy may not be affordable to all and may create even wider socioeconomic differences in future. Citing these reasons, it is prohibited in many countries like India. In certain countries like the UK use may be permitted for mitochondrial disorders after legal permissions. In US trials are governed by Food and Drug Administration (FDA) and National Institute of Health.[3]

■ IN UTERO GENE THERAPY

This modality is still under research on animal models. It is different from germline gene therapy and is a form of somatic cell therapy. It has many advantages. It aims at treating disease in initial stages thereby preventing long-term damage to various organ systems in case of progressive disorders. It has potential to cure in utero lethal disorders. Fetus has plenty of replicating stem cells so there are chances of better efficacy of techniques like CRISPR/cas9 which need replicating cells. Also, the fetus has less blood volume so fewer doses would be needed. The fetus is known to have better immunologic tolerance so the chances of rejection of therapy and toxic immune responses are less. Despite having so many advantages it faces its own set of challenges. Every therapy that is given in utero first should be established to be completely safe to the mother. More research is needed to understand the fetal immunological and neural system which is gestation dependent. More trials would be needed before deciding adequate dose, time of gene therapy, mode of gene delivery and monitoring of mother and fetus after the therapy. Monitoring will also include postnatal surveillance to understand potential of oncogenesis, germline mutation and alteration in immune response and long-term safety. Diseases such as hemoglobinopathies, spinal muscular atrophy, cystic fibrosis, and neurodegenerative disorders are potential candidates for in utero gene therapy.[4]

STRATEGIES OF GENE THERAPY

There are various ways in which gene therapy can be done. There can be either transfer or editing of genetic material.[5] **Flowchart 1** describes strategies of gene therapy.

Genome Editing

A breakthrough research has been the discovery of gene editing tools such as CRISPR/cas9, zinc fingers etc. These systems are capable of causing targeted changes in genome, hence they is more precise, safe, and effective.

APPROACH TO GENE THERAPY

Genetic material cannot be delivered directly into cell nucleus. A carrier or delivery system called vector is generally needed which can transfer DNA inside cell nucleus.[6] There are viral and nonviral vectors. **Flowchart 2** describes types of vectors.

Viral vectors are conventionally used. They are modified in laboratory such that they are able to infect cells and transfer DNA but are unable to produce disease. However, there are certain challenges with use of viral vectors like limitation to the amount of material that can be transferred, they sometime induce exaggerated immune responses which can be life-threatening and stimulate innate immunity making repeated doses ineffective. At times they can also activate oncogenes leading to risk of future cancers. Also, the manufacturing capacity for viral vectors is limited.

To tackle these problems nonviral vectors are being developed but at present they are less effective than viral vectors.

METHODS OF GENE DELIVERY

There can be *ex vivo* or *in vivo* methods of gene delivery.[7] Both therapies have their advantages and disadvantages.

Ex vivo gene therapy: In this therapy, cells from the patient are harvested, transfected with modified virus carrying gene of interest. Virus transfects patient's cells in the laboratory and then these modified cells are amplified and transferred back to the patient. It is mostly applied in hematopoietic stem cells and used to treat blood disorders and immunological disorders. **Figure 1** describes *ex vivo* gene therapy.

In vivo gene therapy: In this, vectors carrying modified genes are injected directly into a patient's systemic circulation or locally. Currently it is used for targeted local therapy like certain retinal dystrophy disorders. Zolgensma for spinal muscular atrophy is also a type of *in vivo* therapy. **Figure 2** describes *in vivo* gene therapy.

HISTORY OF GENE THERAPY

1970s: Potential of gene therapy was recognized.

1980s: Role of viruses as potential vectors was identified.

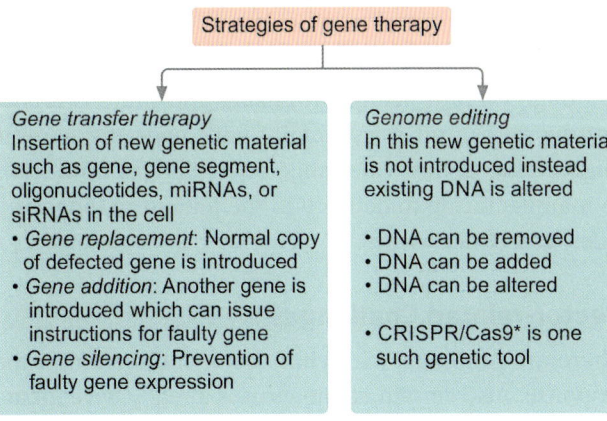

Flowchart 1: Strategies of gene therapy.

*CRISPR/Cas9: Clustered regularly interspaced short palindromic repeats and CRISPR-associated protein 9.

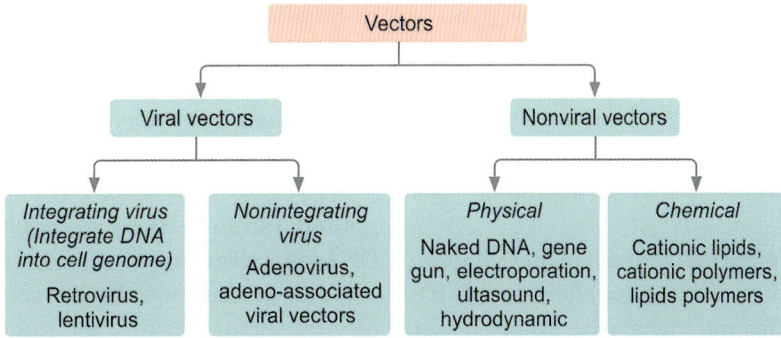

Flowchart 2: Types of vectors.

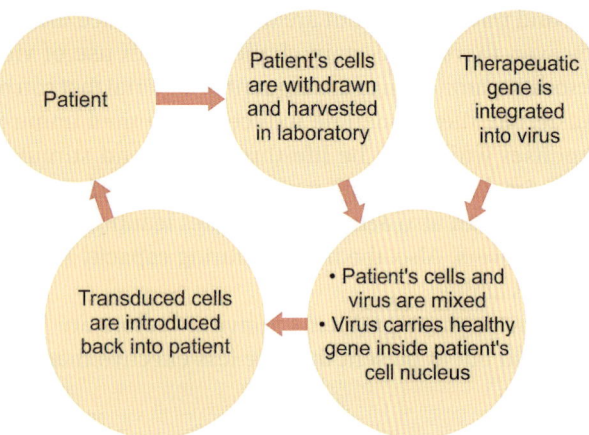

Fig. 1: *Ex vivo* gene therapy.

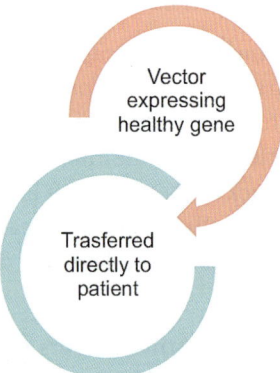

Fig. 2: *In vivo* gene therapy.

1990s: First *ex vivo* gene therapy trial took place.[8,9] It was done in a 4-year-old girl suffering from X-linked severe combined immune deficiency disease. A functioning adenosine deaminase (ADA) gene was transferred in T cells following which levels of T cells normalized and immunity improved. Therapy was based on repeated injections over 2 years but even after discontinuation some effect persisted.[10] This trial gave a lot of promising outlook to gene therapy until two unfortunate incidents happened.

1999: An 18-year-old male was being treated for ornithine transcarbamylase deficiency by adenovirus mediated gene transfer, unfortunately exaggerated immune response led to vector-induced toxicity and multiorgan failure and death.[11]

Later in 2003 it was found that four out of nine children treated for severe combined immunodeficiency (SCID) developed leukemia which was higher than expected rate.

Reason thought was insertional mutagenesis wherein DNA integration can disrupt normally functioning genes and lead to cancers.

These incidents slowed down the pace at which gene therapy trials were going but did not completely stop them. In 2003, Chinese State Food and Drug Administration approved Gendicine for squamous cell carcinoma.[12] 2012, European Medicine Agency (EMA) approved gene therapy product Glybera for treatment of lipoprotein lipase deficiency.[13]

2012: Scientists developed CRISPR/Cas9, a genome editing tool.

2016: EMA-approved Strimvelis for treatment of ADA.

2017: FDA-approved Luxturna for treatment of Leber congenital amaurosis.[14]

2019: FDA-approved Zolgensma for treatment of spinal muscular atrophy.[15]

Over 2,600 clinical trials are underway. We may see several more gene therapies receiving approval in near future.

CHALLENGES WITH GENE THERAPY

Although therapy seems promising and there is lots of optimism around it especially with evolving genetic engineering. It has wide range of challenges from trials to manufacturing to delivery to the patient to long-term safety and ethical issues.[16]

Vector-related Challenges

There are problems with viral vector-induced immune response. Also certain adeno viruses already have innate immunity due to past infections which make gene therapy less effective. New nonviral vectors are being developed but till date they have been found to be less effective.

There are challenges of delivering therapy specifically to target organs. For example, the trials of muscular dystrophy are facing the challenge of delivering drug to the muscle which is a big target organ. Also delivering drug to the central nervous system is challenging due to the blood brain barrier.

There are also long-term safety issues regarding potential of unmasking oncogenes with integration of DNA into cell genome.

A newer challenge that has come up is with the supply of viral vectors. With large number of trials going on and limited manufacturing of viral vectors there is now shortage of supply for trials as well.

Research and Development-related Challenges

Clinical trials for gene therapies being developed for rare disorders face problems with adequate sample size to establish efficacy and safety.

Clinical trials have to be conducted over years to be able to understand long-term effects.

Once the gene therapy is delivered to the patient, its effect cannot be reversed. Unlike drugs where if the effect is no longer desired or there are side effects, drug can be discontinued or other drug can be given to counter the effects.

Manufacturing-related Issues

Only large companies can sustain such lengthy and expensive trials which then translate into commercialization of drug.

There are issues with licensing and patents.

Cost-related Issues

Gene therapy is not only costly to develop but it is costly for patients also to afford. Also there are ethical issues when deciding cost especially when it can be a lifesaving drug to those affected.

Ethical Issues

There are ethical issues regarding safety in human trials, proper monitoring of trials, cost decided by the companies for the drug, balancing commercial motives and humanity, how much gene editing should be ethically allowed as it has potential for misuse as well.

■ CONCLUSION

Gene therapy seems to be a promisable therapy for not only genetic disorders but also for diseases like cancers where no proper treatment is available. With improvement in biotechnology, improvised vectors and gene editing tools we may be able to overcome major challenges like immunogenicity, toxicity, efficacy and oncogenesis. Long-term safety, ethical issues and commercialization are still matters of debate.

■ REFERENCES

1. Gonçalves GAR, Paiva RMA. Gene therapy: advances, challenges and perspectives. Einstein (Sao Paulo). 2017; 15(3):369-75.
2. Nayerossadat N, Maedeh T, Ali PA. Viral and nonviral delivery systems for gene delivery. Adv Biomed Res. 2012;1:27.
3. Liu S. Legal reflections on the case of genome-edited babies. Glob Health Res Policy. 2020;5:24.
4. Peddi N, Marasandra Ramesh H, Gude S, Gude SS, Vuppalapati S, et al. Intrauterine fetal gene therapy: is that the future and is that future now? Cureus. 2022;14(2):e22521.
5. Li H, Yang Y, Hong W, Huang M, Wu M, Zhao X. Applications of genome editing technology in the targeted therapy of human diseases: mechanisms, advances and prospects. Sig Transduct Target Ther. 2020;5(1):1.
6. Razi Soofiyani S, Baradaran B, Lotfipour F, Kazemi T, Mohammadnejad L. Gene therapy, early promises, subsequent problems, and recent breakthroughs. Adv Pharm Bull. 2013;3(2):249-55.
7. Selkirk SM. Gene therapy in clinical medicine. Postgrad Med J. 2004;80(948):560-70.
8. Friedmann T, Roblin R. Gene therapy for human genetic disease? Science. 1972;175(4025):949-55.
9. Williams DA, Lemischka IR, Nathan DG, Mulligan RC. Introduction of new genetic material into pluripotent haematopoietic stem cells of the mouse. Nature. 1984;310(5977):476-80.
10. Blaese RM, Culver KW, Miller AD, Carter CS, Fleisher T, Clerici M, et al. T lymphocyte-directed gene therapy for ADA-SCID: initial trial results after 4 years. Science. 1995;270(5235):475-80.
11. Raper SE, Chirmule N, Lee FS, Wivel NA, Bagg A, Gao GP, et al. Fatal systemic inflammatory syndrome in a ornithine transcarbarmylase deficient patient following adenoviral gene transfer. Mol Genet Metab. 2003;80(1-2): 148-58.
12. Zhang WW, Li L, Li D, Liu J, Li X, Li W, et al., The first approved gene therapy product for Cancer Ad-P53 (Gendicine): 12 years in the clinic. Hum Gene Ther. 2018;29(2):160-79.
13. Liang M. Oncorine, the world first oncolytic virus medicine and its update in China. Curr Cancer Drug Targets. 2018;18 (2):171-6.
14. Padhy SK, Takkar B, Narayanan R, Venkatesh P, Jalali S. Voretigene neparvovec and gene therapy for Leber's congenital amaurosis: review of evidence to date. Appl Clin Genet. 2020;13:179208.
15. Mahajan R. Onasemnogene abeparvovec for spinal muscular atrophy: the costlier drug ever. Int J Appl Basic Med Res. 2019;9 (3):127-8.
16. Kaemmerer WF. How will the field of gene therapy survive its success? Bioeng Transl Med. 2018;3(2):166-77.

INDEX

Page numbers followed by *f* refer to figure, *fc* refer to flowchart, and *t* refer to table

A

Abdomen, fetal 38
Abnormal diagnostic test 23
Achondroplasia 7
Acrocallosal syndrome 38
Adenomatoid malformation, congenital pulmonary 39
Adenomatous polyposis coli 63
Adenosine deaminase 68
Alcohol abuse 38
Alleles 2
Alloimmune thrombocytopenia 19
Alobar holoprosencephaly 36
Alpha-fetoprotein 18, 22, 23
Alpha-plus thalassemia 28, 29
Alpha-thalassemia 28
Alpha-zero thalassemia carrier 28
Amenorrhea, primary 47
American College of Obstetricians and Gynecologists 12
   guidance 12
   recommendations 12
Amniocentesis 17, 18, 19*f*, 24, 61
Amniocyte, failure of 18
Amniotic fluid 18
Androgen insensitivity syndrome 46
Aneuploidy 15, 22, 53, 59
   screening 22
Angelman syndrome 23
Anhydramnios 19
Anorectal anomalies 40
Anorectal atresia 40
Anterior abdominal wall defects 38
Anxiety, low parental 40
Apert syndrome 37
Array comparative genome hybridization 58
Assisted reproductive technologies 58
Ataxia 37
Ataxia-telangiectasia 62
Autosomal dominant disease 5, 64
Autosomal recessive disorder 5, 7, 8*f*, 10, 37
Azoospermia 49
   factor 49
   nonobstructive 48
   obstructive 49

B

Basal cell nevus syndrome 64
Becker muscular dystrophy 11
Beta-galactosidase 11
Beta-thalassemia 28
   major 7, 29
   trait 14
Binder facies 38
   ultrasonography image of 38*f*
Binder syndrome 38, 40
Biochemical marker screening tests 24
Biometric parameters 34
Blake's pouch cyst 36
Blastocyst fluid 60
Blood tests 30
Bloom syndrome 11, 62
Bowel obstruction, prenatal diagnosis of 40
Brain tumors 64
Breast
   cancer 63
      syndrome, hereditary 63
   carcinoma, hereditary 63
   self-examination 64
   tumor of 64
Bronchopulmonary sequestration 39
Buccal mucosa 64

C

Canavan disease 11, 12
Cancer 60
   colorectal 63
   detection 64
   endometrial 64
   hereditary 63*t*
   inherited 62
   peritoneal 50
   predisposition, hereditary 62
   prevention 64
   prostate 63
   renal 63
   syndromes, hereditary nonpolyposis 62, 63, 64*t*
   testicular 50
Cardiac arrhythmia 41
Cardiac rhabdomyoma 41
Cardiovascular diseases 60
Carrier screening 10, 13
Cell-free deoxyribonucleic acid
   detection 17*t*
   test 17
Central nervous system 36
Cephaloceles 37
Cerebellar hypoplasia 37
Chondrodysplasia punctata 38
Chorionic villus sampling 17, 18, 18*f*, 24, 61
Choroid plexus carcinomas 64
Choroid plexus cysts 34
Chromosomal aberrations 38
Chromosomal defects 34
Chromosomal microarray 11, 20, 35, 54
   analysis 24, 34
Chromosomal translocation 54
Chromosome 1
   analysis 11
Cleft lip 38
   nonsyndromic 38
Cleft palate 38
   nonsyndromic 38
Clinical exome sequencing 35
Coloboma 37
Colon polyps 64
Colonoscopy 64
Colorectal cancer, hereditary nonpolyposis 63
Comparative genomic hybridization 54
Complete blood count 12, 29
Comprehensive chromosome screening 58
Copy number variants 3, 20, 22, 54
Cord, free loop of 19
Cordocentesis 18
Corpus callosum, agenesis of 37
Cortical thickness 41
Cowden syndrome 64
Craniotelencephalic dysplasia 37
Cri-du-chat syndrome 23
Cryptorchidism 50
Cyclopia 36
Cystic fibrosis 7, 10, 49, 66
Cystic hygroma 33
Cytotrophoblast cells 60

D

Dandy–Walker malformation 36, 37, 37*f*
Deoxyribonucleic acid 1, 2, 10, 18, 33, 42
   analysis 28
   Biallelic inactivation of 62
   sequences 46
   structure 1*f*
   tests 11
Deoxyribose 2
Diabetes 60
DiGeorge syndrome 20, 33, 41
Double-bubble sign 40
   ultrasonography of 40*f*

Double-cortex syndrome 10
Double-marker test 32
Down syndrome 14, 22, 24, 33, 34
Duchenne muscular dystrophy 9-11, 14
Duodenal atresia 40*f*
Dysautonomia, familial 11

E

Echogenicity 41
Ectrodactyly-ectodermal dysplasia-cleft
    syndrome 38
Embryo transfer 59
Embryogenesis 53
Embryonic aneuploidy 54*f*
Encephalocoele, occipital 37
Endometriosis 47
Endometrium, tumor of 64
Epigenetic studies 55
Estriol, unconjugated 23
Estrogen
    dependent disease 47
    receptor 1 47
Ethmocephaly 36
European Medicine Agency 68
European Society of Human Reproduction
    and Embryology 51
European Urology Association 49
Ex vivo gene therapy 67, 68, 68*f*

F

Fabry disease 10
Facial cleft 33
Facioauriculo vertebral syndrome 37
Fallot's tetralogy 41, 41*f*
Familial cancer syndrome, autosomal
    dominant 64
Fanconi's anemia 11, 40, 58, 62
Female infertility 46
    genetics of 46
Female reproductive system diseases 60
Femur, short length of 34
Fertility preservation 48
Fetal akinesia-deformation sequence 33
Fetal anomalies, congenital 32
Fetal blood 18, 19
    sampling 17-19
Fetal chromosomal microarray 38
Fetal loss 18
    rates 18
Fetal nuchal translucency, sonographic
    determination of 23
Fetal structural abnormalities, universal
    ultrasound screening for 34
Fetal thoracic masses 39
First trimester nuchal translucency 32
Fluorescent in situ hybridization 25, 35,
    49, 58

Follicle-stimulating hormone 47
Food and Drug Administration 66
Fragile X
    mental retardation gene 11, 47
    syndrome 10, 13
Free beta-human chorionic
    gonadotropin 22
Fructose intolerance 11

G

Galactosemia 11
Gametogenesis 46
Gastric cancer 63
    diffuse 63
Gastrointestinal anomalies, fetal 40
Gastrointestinal endoscopy, upper 64
Gastrointestinal tract 63
Gastroschisis 38
Gaucher disease 11
Gene 2
    delivery, methods of 67
    therapy 66-69
        strategies of 67, 67*fc*
        types of 66
Genetics 1, 27, 46, 50, 53, 62
    abnormalities 34
    basics of 1
    carrier testing 10
    counseling 14, 15, 22
    diagnosis, fetal sample for 35*t*
    disorders 14, 42, 66
    inheritance pattern 10
    regulation 30
    role of 46, 50
    sonogram 34
    tests 15, 17, 21, 50
        diagnostic capability of 3*f*
        types of 11, 19
Genitourinary anomalies, fetal 40
Genome 1
    editing 67
Genotype 2
Germ cell 48
    tumor, extragonadal 50
Germline gene therapy 66
Gonadal development 46
Gonadotropin-releasing hormone 47
Gorlin syndrome 64, 65
Gorlin–Goltz syndrome 64
Growth, pulmonary 40
Gynandroblastomas 64

H

Haploinsufficiency 62
Heart
    disease, congenital 41
    fetal 41

Helicobacter pylori infection 63
Hematological malignancies 64
Hematopoietic stem cell transplantation 60
Hemoglobin 27, 28
    electrophoresis 30
    fetal 27
    H disease 29
    normal 27
    types of 28*t*
Hemoglobinopathy 12, 14, 27, 31, 66
    counseling for 30
    screening of 29, 29*fc*
Hemophilia 9, 11, 14
Hemorrhage, fetomaternal 19
Hereditary cancer syndrome, Knudson's
    two-hit hypothesis for 62*f*
Hernia
    congenital diaphragmatic 39
    diaphragmatic 33, 39
    syndromic diaphragmatic 39
Heterozygotes 5
Hexosaminidase, levels of 11
High performance liquid chromatography
    29, 30
High-grade serous adenocarcinoma 63
Histones 1
Hodgkin's lymphoma, hereditary 64
Holoprosencephaly 33, 36, 36*f*
    abortus of 36*f*
Hormones, synthesis of 46
Human chorionic gonadotropin 23, 32, 49
Human leukocyte antigen 59, 60
Human menopausal gonadotropin 48
Humerus, short length of 34
Huntington's disease 7, 10, 60
Hypogonadism
    hypergonadotropic 47
    hypogonadotropic 47, 49
Hypoplasia, lower limb 40
Hypothalamo-pituitary dysfunction 49
Hypoxia 38

I

Ichthyosis 11
Ileum 64
Implantation failure, recurrent 51
In utero gene therapy 66
In vitro fertilization 16, 25, 48, 56, 58
In vivo gene therapy 67, 68*f*
Incontinentia pigmenti 10
Indian Council of Medical Research 14
Infections, perinatal 38
Infertility 46
    female 46
    male 50, 59
Intestinal atresia 40
Intracytoplasmic sperm injection 48
Intrahepatic portal vein, fetal 19

Intrauterine insemination 48
Isochromosomes 55*f*
Isoelectric focusing 29

J

Jacobs syndrome 11
Jejunum 64

K

Kallmann syndrome 47, 49
Karyotype 20, 24, 35
Kearns–Sayre syndrome 59
Klinefelter's syndrome 11, 33, 48
Knudson's two-hit hypothesis 62*f*

L

Lactic acidosis 9
Leber's hereditary optic neuropathy 9, 11
Lesch–Nyhan disease 58
Leukemia, hereditary acute
    lymphoblastic 64
Leydig cell 48
   hypoplasia 49
Li–Fraumeni syndrome 63, 64
Limb-body wall complex 38, 39
Live birth rates 59
Lower small bowel obstructions 40
Lung
   cancer 63
   carcinomas 64
   malformations, congenital 39
Lymphoma 50
Lynch syndrome 63, 64
   genes 63

M

Magnetic resonance imaging 64
   fetal 36
Male infertility 50, 59
   genetics of 48
Malnutrition 38
Maple syrup urine disease 11
Marfan syndrome 7, 10
Mastectomy 64
Maxillofacial dysplasia 38
Mayer–Rokitansky–Kuster–Hauser
    syndrome 46
Mean corpuscular
   hemoglobin 28, 29
   volume 29, 30
Meckel–Gruber syndrome 37
Medullary thyroid carcinoma 64
Medulloblastoma 64
Megacystis 41
   microcolon intestinal hypoperistalsis
    syndrome 41

Melanoma 63
Mendelian syndrome 38
Metabolic disorders, inborn errors of 11
Metabolism, inborn errors of 14, 38
Methylation 3
Microdeletions 24
   syndromes 40
Mitochondrial deoxyribonucleic acid 60
Mitochondrial encephalopathy 9, 11
Mitochondrial inheritance 5, 9, 9*f*, 11
Molecular testing 38
Monogenic disorders 59
Monosomy 46, 53
Mosaicism 3, 54
Mucolipidosis 11
Müllerian anomalies 46, 48
Multicystic kidney disease 41
Multifactorial disorders 66
Multiple endocrine neoplasia 62, 64
Multiple gastrointestinal hamartomatous
    polyps 64
Multiple marker serum-only test 23
Multiplex ligation-dependent probe
    amplification 35
   analysis 30

N

Nasal bone 33*f*
Nephroblastoma 64
Neural tube defects 22
Neurodegenerative disorders 66
Neurofibromatosis 20, 64, 65
Neurosonogram 36
Nevoid basal cell carcinoma syndrome 64
Next-generation sequencing 11, 20, 37, 42,
   48, 58
Niemann–Pick disease 11
Nijmegen breakage syndrome 62
Noninvasive preimplantation genetic
    testing 60
Noninvasive prenatal screening 17
Nonmendelian inheritance 9
Noonan syndrome 33
Nuchal fold thickness 34*f*
Nuchal translucency 32, 32*f*

O

Oculoencephalohepato-renal syndrome 37
Oligohydramnios 40, 41
Oligophrenia 37, 49
Omphalocele 38, 39, 39*f*
Oncogenes 62
Orphan diseases 14
Osteosarcomas 64
Ovarian cancer 63
   hereditary 63
   screening 64
   syndrome, hereditary 63
Ovarian carcinoma, hereditary 63

P

Pancreatic cancer 63
Pancreatic islet cells 64
Parathyroid glands 64
Pedigree 5
   analysis of 5, 9
   chart 5, 7*f*, 8*f*
   symbols 7*f*
    standard 6*f*
Pelviureteric junction obstruction 40
Peripheral blood karyotype 48
Peutz–Jeghers syndrome 64
Phenotype 2
Phenylketonuria 11, 38
Pheochromocytoma 64
Pigmentations, mucocutaneous 64
Placental cord insertion site 19
Placental growth factor 23
Plasma protein-A, pregnancy-associated
   18, 22, 23, 32
Pleiotropy 3
Pleuropulmonary blastomas 64
Polycystic kidney, autosomal dominant 41
Polycystic ovary syndrome 47
Polygenic disease 60
Polyhydramnios 40
Polymerase chain reaction 18, 36
Polymorphisms 2, 56
Polyposis syndrome 63
Posterior fossa cystic lesions 36
Prader–Willi syndrome 23
Preconception genetic counseling 14
Pregnancy 53
   loss 53
    recurrent 50, 53, 56
    repeated 59
   maintenance 55
   termination of 23
   twin 24
Preimplantation genetic
   diagnosis 15, 50, 56, 58
   screening 15, 56, 58
   testing 49, 50, 58-60
    indications for 59
Premature ovarian insufficiency 46, 47
Prenatal genetic testing, indications of 19
Prenatal serum screening 23
PTEN hamartoma tumor syndrome 64
Pyelectasis 34, 41

Q

Quadruple marker test 23
Quantitative fluorescence polymerase chain
    reaction 25, 35
Quantitative real-time polymerase chain
    reaction 58

R

Randomized controlled trial 58
Rapamycin, mammalian target of 65
Red-green color blindness 9, 10
Renal agenesis 41
Renal cell carcinomas 65
Renal disorders 41
Retinal dystrophy disorders 67
Retinoblastoma 64
Rett syndrome 10
Rhabdomyosarcomas 64
Ribonucleic acid 11
Ring chromosome 55*f*
Robertsonian translocations 11, 55*f*, 59

S

Sacral agenesis 40
Sandhoff disease 11
Sanger sequencing 35
Sarcomas 64
Sclerosis, tuberous 65
Screening tests, types of 23
Screen-positive cell-free DNA-based test 24
Second trimester genetic sonogram 33
Seizures 41
Sertoli–Leydig cell tumors 64
Serum screening 22
    abnormal 22
Sex chromosome 49
    abnormalities 48
    aneuploidy 17
Sexual development
    disorders of 49
    female 46
Sickle cell
    anemia 7, 10, 14, 22, 27, 28
    disease 12, 30
    trait 28
Sickle hemoglobin 27
Single gene disorder 37*f*, 39, 50
Single nucleotide
    polymorphism 55
        testing 58
    variant 2
Skeletal disorders 40

Skeletal dysplasia 14, 40
Skeletal system 40
Skewed X chromosome inactivation 55
Skin, tumor of 64
Soft tissue sarcomas 64
Somatic gene therapy 66
Spermatogenetic failure 49
Spinal muscular atrophy 12, 14, 66
Stomach 64
Swyer syndrome 46

T

Tay-Sachs disease 7, 10-12
Teratozoospermia, severe 59
Testicular dysgenesis syndrome 50
Testicular failure 48
Testicular germ cell tumor 50
Testicular microlithiasis 50
Testicular sperm extraction 48
Tetraploidy 53
Thalassemia 11, 27, 28, 30*f*
    carrier 30*f*
    intermedia 29
    major 29
    minor 29
    screening 30
Thyroid, tumor of 64
Toxoplasmosis, rubella, cytomegalovirus, and herpes simplex virus 36
Transcerebellar plane 34
Transforming growth factor beta 47
Transvaginal ultrasound examination 64
Trinucleotide repeat expansion 3
Trio exome sequencing 35
Triploidy 53
Trisomy 17, 33*f*, 53
Trophoblast culture, failure of 18
Trophoblastic cells 17
Tumor
    colon 64
    hereditary 64
    kidney 64
    pediatric 64
    suppressor gene 62, 63
Turner's syndrome 11, 33, 38, 41, 46, 48, 49, 58

U

Ultrasound 32
    abnormalities 33
    scan 18*f*
Urinary tract dilatation 40
    disorders 40

V

VACTERL syndrome 40
Van der Woude syndrome 38
Vas deferens, congenital bilateral absence of 49
Vectors, types of 67*fc*
Velocardiofacial syndrome 33
Ventricular septal defects 41
Ventriculomegaly 33, 36
Viral vectors 67
von Hippel–Lindau syndrome 65

W

Walker Warburg syndrome 37
Whole exome sequencing 20, 35, 48, 54
Whole genome sequencing 21, 35
Wilms' tumor 64
Wolf–Hirschhorn syndrome 38
Worsening 41

X

X chromosome 46, 48
X-linked dominant disorders 10
X-linked recessive disorders 10
XX gonadal dysgenesis 47
XY gonadal dysgenesis 46

Y

Y chromosome 48
    cluster mutation 49
    microdeletion 49
Y-linked disorders 5, 9

Z

Zona pellucida 47
    formation of 47